The Rhythm of Rescue

A CPR History and Memoir

Monica Stephens

Internet addresses given in this book were accurate at the time it went to press.

This book is intended as a reference volume only, not as a medical manual. The information given here is designed to inspire and inform. It is not intended as a substitute for any treatment that may have been prescribed by your doctor. If you suspect that you have a medical problem, we urge you to seek competent medical help.

The personal stories presented here are their own recollections and memories. They have done their best to be faithful to their experiences, but memory is imperfect. They have also done their best to present other people in the most positive lights. These stories are printed here with permission.

Printed in the United States of America
Published in Hellertown, PA

Cover design by Leanne Coppola
ISBN paperback: 979-8-89420-104-7
ISBN hardcover: 979-8-89420-105-4
Library of Congress Control Number 2026911275

For more information or to place bulk orders, contact the author or the publisher at Jennifer@BrightCommunications.net.

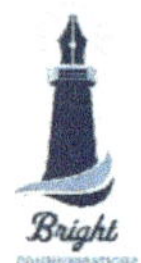

To my Rubix Cube who gave me my love of books
and to my mother to avoid any possible jealousy LOL

Contents

Foreword

When Monica asked me to write the foreword for this book, I was genuinely honored.

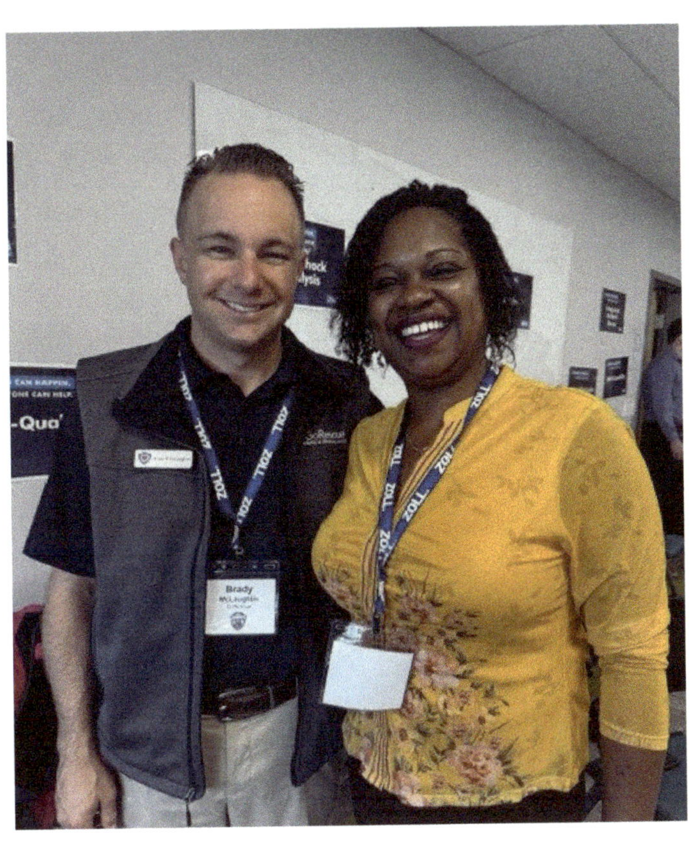

Not simply because I know how much work goes into writing a book, but because this one matters.

For years, those of us in the CPR+AED world have lived inside an industry that most people only think about during an emergency, after a tragedy, or when they need a certification card for work. But behind the scenes, an entire movement of people has dedicated their lives to helping others survive sudden cardiac arrest.

This book captures that.

I have never ever seen someone bring together the history, heart, innovation, entrepreneurship, science, and humanity of the modern CPR+AED movement quite like Monica has done here.

And the reason she was able to do it so well is simple: She lives it.

Monica is not writing from a distance. She understands what it means to teach the classes, build the programs, serve the customers, support the survivors, solve the problems, and continue showing up because you believe lives can be saved if people are simply prepared.

This resonates deeply with me.

Years ago, my wife and I launched our CPR+AED company because of a question God placed on our hearts: *How do we help save more lives outside the context of working a shift as a first responder?*

The answer became clear: *Train and equip people. And do it at scale.*

That mission changed our lives.

Many people outside of this industry do not fully realize the amount of effort, intentionality, detail, and energy that go into every CPR class and every AED program. The public sees a CPR card or an AED on a wall. What they often do not see are the countless hours, planning, retraining, compliance efforts, medical oversight, quality assurance, readiness checks, follow-up, advocacy, and passion behind it all.

All of it exists for one reason: *To give someone the absolute best chance of survival on the worst day of their life.*

That is why this work matters.

And that is why this book matters.

As I read these pages, I found myself reflecting on the history of CPR and AEDs and also on the people who helped build this movement—the instructors, survivors, manufacturers, entrepreneurs, healthcare providers, first responders, innovators, and advocates who truly believe ordinary people can save lives.

Because they can.

One thing I hope readers take away from this book is that we still have so much work to do. The largest number of sudden cardiac arrests outside the hospital still happen in the home— ground zero—yet CPR training and AEDs are still far from common in American homes.

That MUST change.

My prayer is that this book sparks something.

Maybe it encourages someone to finally attend a CPR class.

Maybe a family decides to purchase an AED.

Maybe a survivor finds the courage to tell their story.

Maybe a future instructor or entrepreneur discovers their calling in this industry.

Maybe someone simply walks away with a greater appreciation for the people working every day to strengthen the chain of survival.

I believe Monica—via this very book in your hands—will help move that mission forward.

She has done an incredible job preserving the history of this industry while also capturing the passion that continues to drive it into the future.

And for that, I am grateful.

—Brady B. McLaughlin, MS, NREMT

Cofounder, GoRescue Brands, LLC (a Safe Life Company)

Lifesaving Leadership Advocate

Introduction

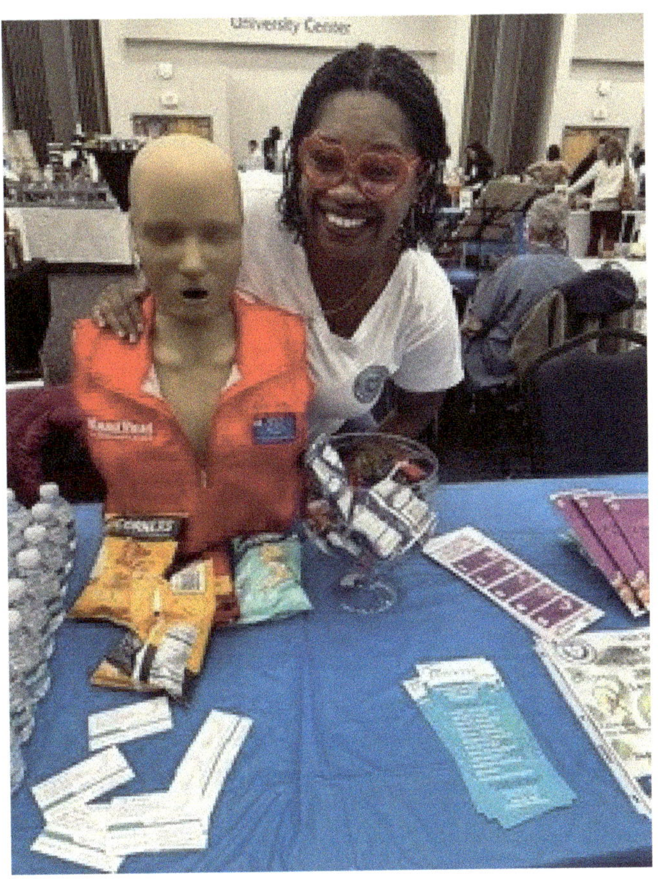

As a CPR and first aid educator, I must deliver engaging classes that empower each of my students to save a life when needed. All the tools and techniques I share in my classes build confidence, which can make the difference between action and inaction, between a life saved and a life lost.

Maybe it's the journalist in me, the educator, or both, but I had a lot of questions about the history of CPR, including.

How did we get to this point in CPR education?

How did we develop the tools that we have to teach CPR?

Why should people care enough to learn CPR?

Wait! How do we even have CPR?

When I launched my podcast, the Wellness Pulse, in 2025, I discovered that many people both inside the CPR instruction community and beyond were also curious about the history of CPR.

I began to reflect upon my own journey through CPR education, where I have met so many other genius entrepreneurs, and I couldn't help but reminisce. I have been teaching CPR for more than 15 years. When I first began teaching, there were not many other instructors. Those few instructors were not necessarily entrepreneurs, and even if they were, they weren't typically forthcoming with knowledge.

My mother, a seasoned registered respiratory therapist and I founded People's Choice CPR in Groveport, Ohio, in 2009. By the spring of 2010, I became a Basic Life Support (BLS) instructor. That summer I went on vacation to Florida and never left. Yes, I took my manikins and ran for the beach!

I found myself in Florida after a failed marriage and in a faltering career, both of which called me to do something fulfilling, something worthwhile. The Lord always said that you should love your neighbor like yourself, right? I know if I experienced sudden cardiac arrest, I would want someone to help me, but what if they didn't know how?

Teaching people how to perform CPR seemed like the right thing to do because the best way to love someone is to teach them how to save their loved ones! I began teaching classes on the beach—and attracting a lot of attention with my PRESTAN manikins that light up! I felt empowered and confident as an educator.

As I began teaching CPR classes in Florida, my mother continued teaching in Ohio. Despite the new distance between us, we continued to work close together to provide high-quality classes that gave participants the confidence to perform lifesaving CPR. We dressed baby manikins in sleepers and adult manikins in T-shirts to simulate a more life-like environment. We brought up sensitive subjects, such as what to do if a victim is a woman or has large breasts.

As I continued my life path, I embarked on becoming a registered nurse in 2012. My background in journalism and psychology contributed to my desire to provide high-quality information and class delivery. I truly believe that knowledge is power, and I take education very seriously.

After I graduated from nursing school, People's Choice CPR struggled to expand. My customers were mainly repeat business and referrals, but we weren't growing. My mother, whose philosophy is "flexible is good," researched new business options and learned about GoRescue, an American Heart Association CPR Training Center that assisted instructors with certifications and business functions through partnership and collaboration. We attended their fifth annual Lifesaving Summit, where I was impressed by the growth of MCR Medical and PRESTAN. (More on these companies in Chapters 7, 8, and 9.)

The educational sessions, presentations, and networking at the Lifesaving Summit blew my mind. I was delighted to meet so many entrepreneurs and humbled by their welcome. I learned a lot about new CPR products, and I was impressed with the variety of options.

Over the next few years, I worked to grow and improve my business to be able to help more people learn the lifesaving skill of CPR. It occurred to me that I wanted to do something to pay homage to CPR and to propel the CPR industry forward. Granted, I teach high-quality CPR, but I wanted to do something more.

I realized I could inform and inspire many more people than can attend my classes with a podcast, so I launched the Wellness Pulse. I wanted to teach people that CPR isn't just a training or job requirement. It's an act of love. It could be what saves your friend, your loved one, or yourself.

For my podcast, I spoke with many wonderful people in the CPR community. I also spoke with survivors. The more I learned about the history and stories of CPR, the more I wanted to share with others. So join me on this super fun stroll through *The Rhythm of Rescue: A CPR History and Memoir.*

Chapter 1: Before the Beat Began

Scan to learn more about CPR history.

As I grew into my journey to answer the question *Where did CPR even come from*? I realized I didn't know much about the history of CPR. To be honest, I taught for years without really pondering the history of CPR, so then I wondered what made me wonder that all of a sudden. Perhaps it's because I spend so much time trying to make sure that I convey the proper techniques and empower people to save lives. Maybe it's because I do not understand why everyone doesn't prioritize learning CPR as highly as I do. Possibly, it's just how I am. I thought that perhaps if people could get to know the CPR advocates, instructors, businesses and their "why," we could connect on the human aspect. Let's learn CPR, for whatever reason, even if it's sentimental. I wanted to know: *Who are these CPR instructors? Better yet, who are these survivors?*

I was convinced that CPR was born out of desperation, the desperate wanting to preserve another human being. It turns out I was right. CPR *was* born out of desperation, but the history of CPR is filled with many tales, many desperations that converged together.

Early efforts to resuscitate people were creative, but chaotic. It wasn't until the mid-20th century that CPR finally combined oxygen delivery and blood circulation based on then-current science. It has saved—and continues to save—millions of lives ever since. Today's CPR is the result of centuries of heart and hope, and a lot of trial and error.

For me, this Bible verse is kind of where everything starts.

"And the LORD God formed man of the dust of the ground, and breathed into his nostrils the breath of life; and man became a living soul."—Genesis 2:7 (KJV)

However, it is important to note that the Bible was not compiled until thousands of years after these occurrences. These accounts most likely circulated verbally until the various scholars recorded their works in their religious texts, including the Christian Bible (I referenced the King James Version), the Tanakh (Hebrew Bible), the Qur'an (Islamic Sacred text), African Christian Biblical canons, and others.

> I was convinced that CPR was born out of desperation, the desperate wanting to preserve another human being.

Seemingly, the idea that breath equated life was an accepted understanding.

The inner workings of what allowed man to live were another skill set of understanding. I say that because people innately seem to know that a

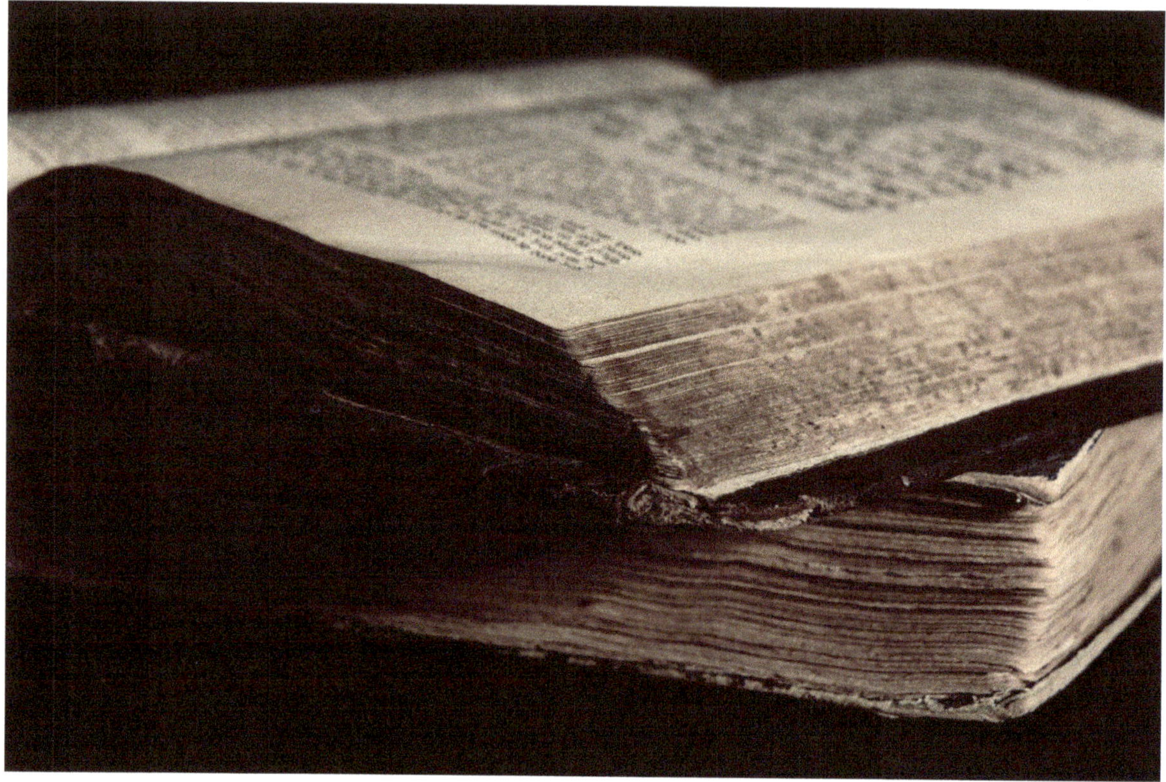

non-breathing person did not have life. They were typically cold to the touch—or at least colder than a breathing person.

People realized we need to warm the body and make it breathe again. Back then, the medical knowledge was intermingled with spiritual and religious knowledge. Honestly, this is still the case for many of us. Today, we have science to better understand the inner workings of why humans live, but I know when someone needs CPR, a lot of us are praying! It took a while for people to rely on scientific processes, and up until then a lot of medical practices incorporated divinity.

Another account from the Christian Bible that can be viewed as early emergency medical treatment is in the first book of Kings 17:21-23 (KJV).

"And he stretched himself upon the child three times, and cried unto the LORD, and said, O LORD my God, I pray thee, let this child's soul come into him again. And the LORD heard the voice of Elijah; and the soul of the child came into him again and he revived."

This scripture isn't as cut and dry, but if you envision this in your mind, you definitely see the child taking in a breath when revived. I do not know what scientifically we can compare to "stretching oneself upon the child." Maybe compression? I know I am kind of reaching on that one.

My final Christian Biblical reference is Second Kings 4:34 (KJV), where Elisha basically performed mouth-to-resuscitation and treated shock with the knowledge of the age.

"And he went up, and lay upon the child, and put his mouth upon his mouth, and his eyes upon his eyes, and his hands upon his hands, and he stretched himself upon the child; and the flesh of the child waxed warm."

Of course, all of these Biblical examples were written to showcase miracles, not CPR, but one can see how Bible readers would have been curious about these treatments. Maybe they even mimicked them to try to understand how to revive people.

I suppose that in Biblical times drowning was a common cause of near deaths and a common medical emergency of the time. There seems to be a lot of instruction relating to drowning/near-drowning as the main medical emergency. Those are the conclusions I deduced anyway.

Ideas and practices like that must have circulated among the spiritual and medical providers of different cultures and regions. Ancient Greek and Roman physicians such as Galen used reed-to-mouth instruments to blow air into the lungs of dead animals, proving that air inflates the lungs when introduced to the area. Galen experimented on different animals, such as pigs, monkeys, apes, goats, sheep, and dogs.

Pretty much up until about 600-700 AD, people around the world did many different things to treat cardiopulmonary arrest. Because they didn't really know what it was, they likely prayed and used whatever medicinal practices they had available, such as aromatics and herbs, applying pressure or rubbing, managing temperature, and body positioning. This could have included lying the person in a flat position, lying them on their side to prevent choking or to manage secretions, elevating their head, and even turning or repositioning the body. Likely, people combined those practices.

After that time, Christian medical compositions (writings about medicinal work, including descriptions of anatomy, treatments, observations, or instructions) began to surface. Some were translated into Arabic during the Islamic Golden Age, which was a time of Islamic Empire expansion with an emphasis on learning. Advancements in medicine, science, and philosophy were encouraged and even state-funded. There were organized translations of Greek medical texts, like those of Galen and Hippocrates, into Arabic. Simultaneously, people in China were making medical advancements, documenting their findings, and creating protocols. Documented advancements continued throughout Persia and Syria/Egypt.

In 1258 AD, during what is regularly referred to as the "Sack of Baghdad," much of this medical knowledge of the Islamic Golden Age was damaged or destroyed. Baghdad, a major political and cultural center of the Abbasid empire, was taken by Mongol forces led by Hulagu Khan during the rule of Al-Musta'sim. Many libraries and hospitals and even scholars were lost, which slowed the momentum of progress. The city's fall led to the rapid collapse of its civic and scholarly infrastructure, including libraries, teaching centers, and systems that supported medical learning and practice. Contemporary accounts describe the destruction of manuscripts on a massive scale. Some books written since describing the event were illustrated with an image of the Tigris River darkened with ink—capturing the depth of intellectual disruption, whether taken literally or as metaphor.

Consequently, for a few hundred years, much of the world experienced stagnation in the development of the healing arts. From that time, there is not a lot of documented experimental research. Anatomical progression slowed, and no systematic revival techniques were established. Religious doctrine was still there, and the idea that breathing equated life remained. Conceivably, many healers relied on prayer, aromatics, possibly pressure application, and quirky stimulation techniques like flagellation.

If I am being completely transparent, it is hard for me to understand the vastness of the super powers of that time. Times were so different, as were their priorities and even the way knowledge was discovered and shared. It is hard to say what Spain, Portugal, France, England, the Ottoman Empire, the Ming Dynasty, the Mughal Empire, the Safavid Empire, Songhai Empire, and Ethiopia were doing regarding resuscitation at that time, not to mention, the smaller regional pockets. There might have been some obscure resuscitation practices used back then that despite my sincerest efforts, I did not uncover.

Before the development of modern sciences, religious beliefs often inspired medical advancements and treatments and were intermingled with cultural histories. Illness was often explained through spiritual influences, divine will, and religious balance theories. The people who had advanced knowledge that enabled other people to survive used it.

Concerning resuscitation knowledge, the 1500s saw the advent of resuscitation knowledge with a process called the Bellows Method. People had used bellows for non-medicinal purposes since the Bronze Age. Different regions of the world independently created their own bellows to control or enhance fires and in metallurgy. Bellows control heat by increasing air flow. When the bellows is expanded, it draws air in, and when the bellows is compressed, the air is forced out.

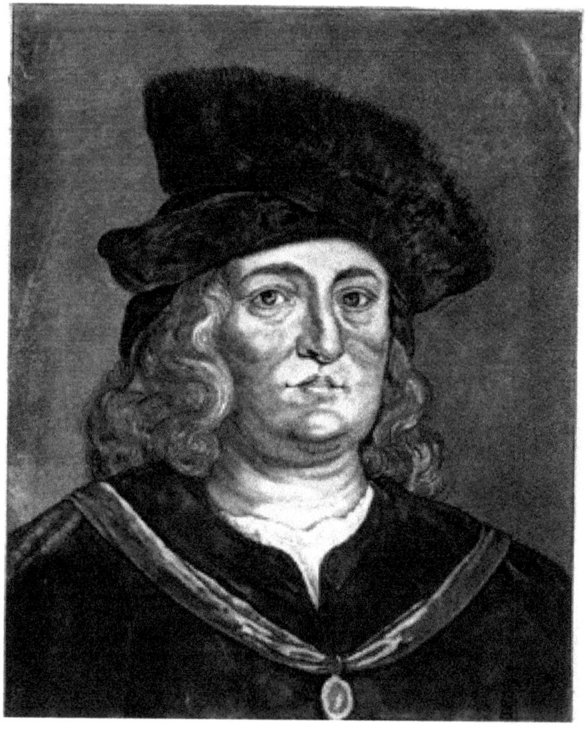

The bellow's development as a medical intervention is credited to a Swiss physician known as Paracelsus. I truly enjoyed reading about this guy. He seemed like quite the character!

Paracelsus was born Philippus Aureolus Theophrastus Bombastus von Hohenheim in Einsiedeln, Switzerland. His father, Wilhelm Bombast von Hohenheim, was a physician, chemist, and minor nobleman. Probably because Philippus's birth name was quite a mouthful, he renamed himself "Paracelsus," which is Latinized "beyond Celsus." Celsius was a classical Roman medical big dog, so pretty much Philippus was saying he was beyond ancient medicine. He was described as a physician, alchemist, philosopher, and medical reformer.

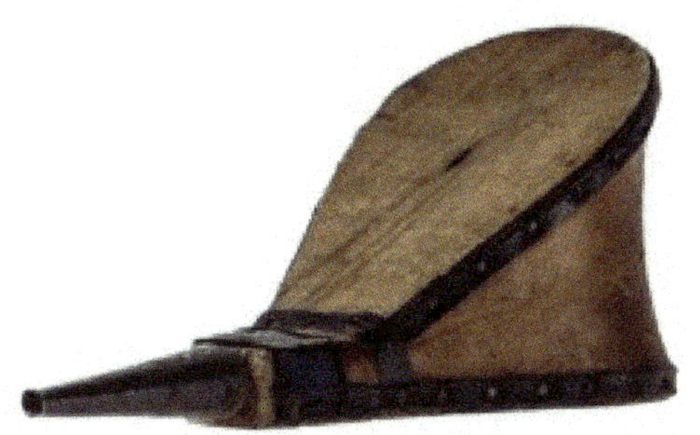

Paracelsus's father had Latinized the surname from Bombast to Bombastus. (Fun fact, it was common to Latinize names during that era.) Paracelsus's mother's vocation was lost to history. It is plausible that she was a bondswoman, hospital stewardess, or nurse. She died during Paracelsus's youth. The family was middle to upper-middle class. They lived modestly, and they had to move for Wilhelm to work. Hence, Paracelsus had access to education and exposure to various geographical areas, books, mining, traditional and folk medicine, surgery and treatments for injuries, metal ores, alchemy, and chemistry.

Why bellows? I imagine that through all of Paracelsus's experiences, bellows must have resonated as a tool that could assist in reversing respiratory failure by forcing air into the lungs.

Although the Bellows Method was a revolutionary idea at the time and advanced lifesaving science, it didn't likely save very many people. Historical accounts suggest that many people who received the Bellows Method were already dead—long passed the point of resuscitation, possibly even decomposing. Some of the resurrection stories involve people being dead for days, then revived, and those stories cast doubt on whether or not any of the Bellows Method attempts were actually successful.

Plus, the Bellows Method was kind of dangerous. The amount of air being forced into a patient's lungs could cause damage to their mouth, lungs, and alveoli.

As a medical reformer, Paracelsus challenged ancient teachings that were accepted as truth, believing that machines or technology could assist with sustaining life. He's described as anti-establishment, anti-university orthodoxy, and also aggressively self-promoting. He knew he was revolutionary, and he acted the part. As his given name was Bombastus, some people called him "bombastic" with his arrogant, loud, theatrical ways. He caused quite a stir within the straight-laced academia, even gaining some enemies. He bad-mouthed other physicians, publicly burned traditional medical books, and practiced folk medicine and alchemy. He continued to move often, living a very nomadic life and never marrying or having any known children.

At least two unfavorable or very biased biographies that were written about Paracelsus reported that he abused alcohol. Later, he became known as the father of toxicology. He denounced the popular medical opinion at the time that illness was caused by an imbalance of humours in the body. Instead, he theorized illness was due to toxins or a system imbalance.

Paracelsus's methods were precursors to experimental science. He wanted to see things in practice, a proto-modern physician, which is a medical practitioner from the transitional period between traditional and modern medicine, someone who began applying systematic observation, anatomy, and early scientific methods to healthcare and helped shift toward evidence-based practice. Although Paracelsus wasn't always liked or agreed with, he did make people think. He seemed like a real "to know him is to love him or hate him" kind of guy. Ironically, he was more appreciated after his death.

At some point, the Bellows Method transitioned from *oral* therapy to *anal* therapy. This might have been because of the risk of lung damage when air was forced into the mouth. Later, forcing oxygen into the body was replaced by forcing tobacco smoke into the body with bellows. This caused a variety of injuries, including burns, perforation, and sepsis.

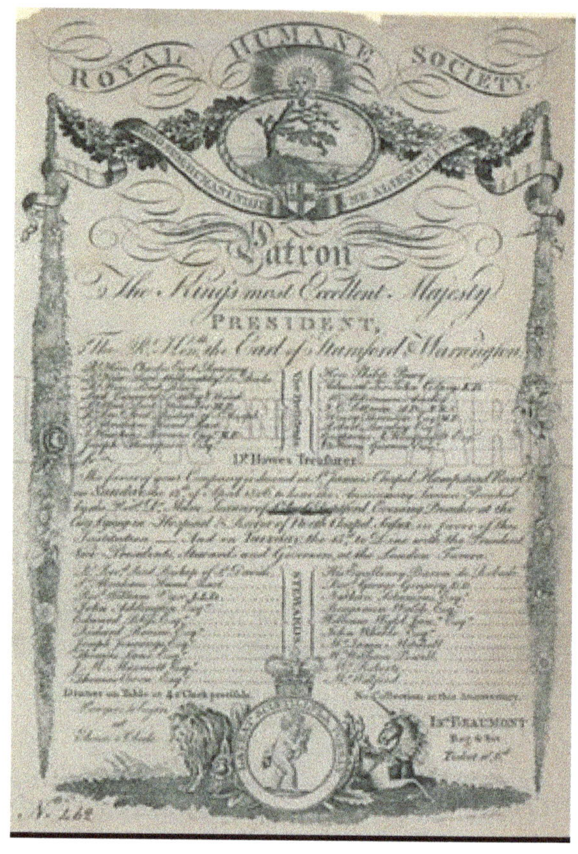

Research is unclear, but it points to tobacco smoke first being used by North American Native Americans or First Nations Peoples in medicinal, spiritual, and ceremonial purposes. Some Indigenous peoples even used tobacco enemas for religious or other health issues, but not for resuscitation.

The practice became accepted in European culture. In the 1700s, the use of tobacco smoke enemas was believed to reheat and stimulate organs. This was actually condoned by the Royal Humane Society back in the 1700s and 1800s, which promoted tobacco smoke enemas to revive drowning victims. By 1767, the Royal Humane Society had ordained tobacco smoke enema kits as an emergency revival procedure.

Tobacco smoke was blown into the patient's rectum using a bellows and a tube inserted into the patient. Some physicians even used long-stemmed pipes to blow the smoke by mouth. The belief was that nicotine and heat would stimulate respiration, warm the body, and potentially save the life. The rectum was chosen because it was believed to absorb stimulants quickly into the bloodstream. Back then, enemas were commonly used for medicine delivery, so this likely felt right to people at that time based on their science and medical views.

In my opinion, some of these medical views are mixed with spiritual connotations from various cultures and timeframes. Reviving the spirit or the human essence was spiritual, so initial resuscitation techniques might have been about doing something to the spirit or soul.

Tobacco smoke enema kits were even stationed along the Thames River in London for emergency use. However, there are no confirmed, scientifically documented cases of tobacco smoke enemas successfully reviving anyone from drowning or cardiac arrest. In rare cases, a person who was only hypothermic might have woken up, but that had nothing to do with the tobacco itself.

Tobacco smoke enema kits were even stationed along the Thames River in London for emergency use.

In the end, the Royal Humane Society helped legitimize the public's lifesaving efforts, even if some of their methods were off or misguided related to today's science. And the phrase "blow smoke up your arse" originated from this practice. Today, we use that expression to describe false flattery or insincere praise.

The Royal Humane Society Poster Resuscitation Steps

- *Remove from water*
- *Dry and warm the body*
- *Blow air into the lungs*
- *Manipulate chest/abdomen*
- *Stimulate the body*
- *Continue for hours if needed*

The Tobacco Smoke Enema Kits
How It Was Done

- *A bellow would push smoke through a canister and into a rectal tube inserted into the patient.*
- *Some physicians elected to use long stemmed pipes to blow the smoke by mouth.*
- *The rectum was selected for quicker stimulant absorption into the bloodstream.*
- *The kits were stationed along the River Thames in London, for emergency use.*

With their smoke enema kits placed along the river for public use, the Royal Humane Society helped to standardize resuscitation and provide the first public protocol for reviving the dead. They even made rescuing people in need a civil duty by training the public and paying rescuers. They solidified mouth-to-mouth in the history books. This is important because although it fell out of favor, it would resurface in the 1950s.

If you are like me, you are wondering, who was actually doling out tobacco smoke enemas? It turns out physicians, barber-surgeons/surgeons, medical students and apprentices, apothecary workers, resuscitation society volunteers, and lay rescuers such as river workers, fishermen, boatmen, police, and bystanders trained with pamphlets. If people were willing to blow smoke into someone's tush, doing CPR should be no problem.

Other less invasive fumigation practices at that time aimed to revive people might have involved burning herbs, such as frankincense, myrrh, rosemary, and sage, or boiling vinegar to make a vapor near a patient, creating a smoke bath.

Around the 1800-1820s, once medical thinking and mainstream society came to the conclusion that tobacco smoke was not good for people, tobacco smoke treatments became obsolete. Meanwhile, other healers were hanging unresponsive people upside down, rolling them on barrels, and placing them on trotting horses to try to revive them. I hope they were secured and placed upon a horse that listened!

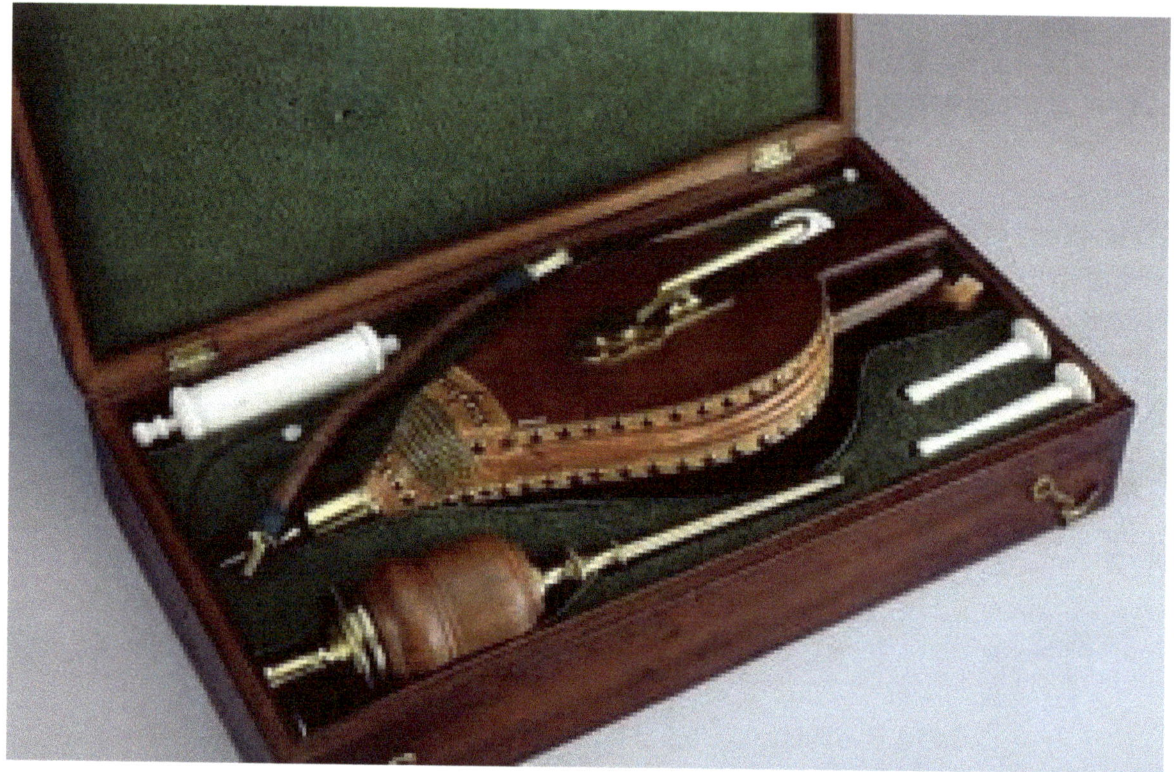

We should take a stroll now down biopiracy lane. It's only right to point out that many explorers and conquerors acquired Indigenous knowledge of biological resources without consent or compensation, maybe even deceptively. The intellectual theft occurred all the time, all over the world.

Early Indigenous resuscitation ideas, including breath stimulation, heat therapy, tobacco pharmacology (as mentioned previously) and ritual revival practices, were quite conceivably observed by explorers and conquerors, and the practices very well could have been misunderstood or altered to be institutionalized by Europeans.

England, France, the Netherlands and Spain contributed the most to colonial medical records in the Americas while Portugal produced the largest quantity in Brazil and extensive regions of Africa and Asia.

Breath stimulation practices included the use of tobacco smoke as previously discussed, and also by less invasive methods like burning the smoke in the vicinity of the person or directing the smoke toward them. Heat therapies included placing patients close to a fire, wrapping them in blankets or coverings, placing warmed stones near them, and steam/sweat exposure to gradually rewarm the body.

The term "folk medicine" often refers to medicine that people acquired from Indigenous people, rebranded as their own science, and omitted the actual people who created it.

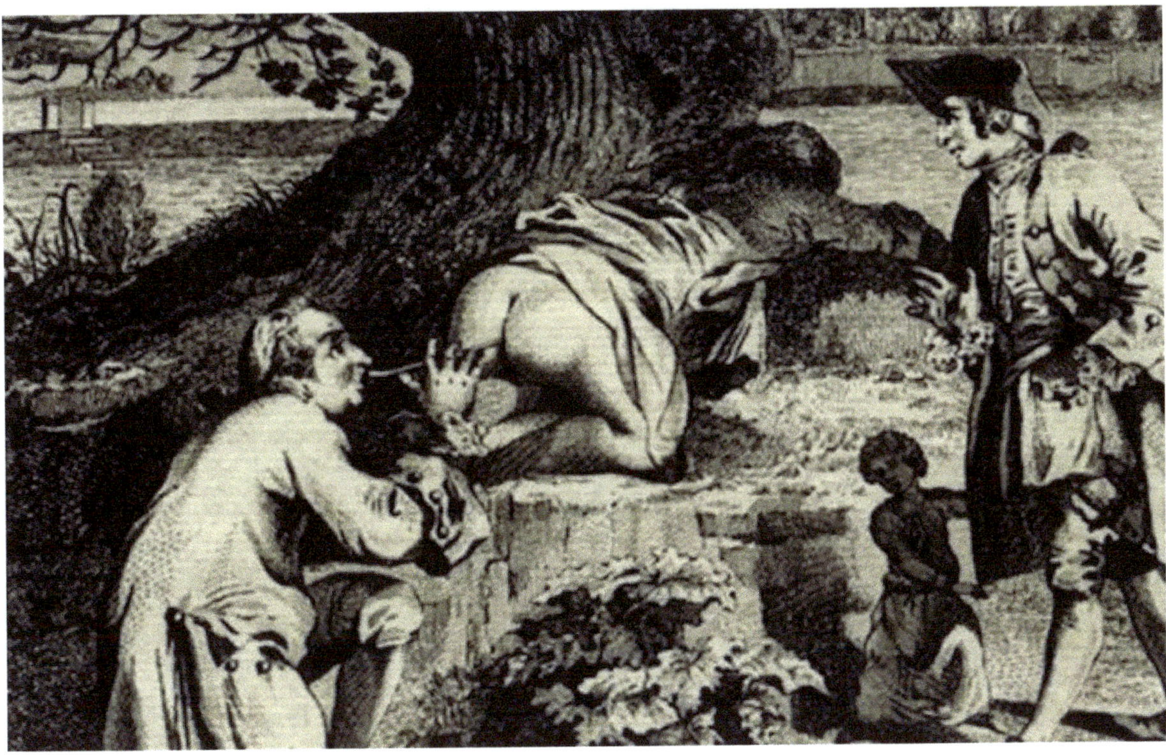

In 1856, the science of lifesaving really started to take form when Marshall Hall fathered the "Ready Method," which is also named for him as the "Hall Method." Marshall Hall was an English physician and physiologist whose work on reflexes and the nervous system inspired further understanding of life and revival. He was born in England when medicine was shifting from tradition-based to science-based. He studied at the University of Edinburgh, which was one of the leading medical schools of the time. He trained in classical medicine, anatomy, and early physiology. His work focused on how the body responded automatically to stimuli, and he was one of the first to describe what we now call reflex function. He helped establish the concept of automatic nervous system responses, the reflex arc.

Hall explored how breathing and reflexes relate to survival. This curiosity laid the foundation for his work on resuscitation methods later in his career. First, a non-responsive victim would be placed prone to allow water and any bodily fluids to expel themselves out of the mouth. This method was the first to hone in on the importance of draining fluid from the airway: the first known step in building our current airway management protocols. Then the victim would be turned onto their side, then their back, then their other side, then to their stomach, over and over, 12 to 15 rolls per minute. These movements created chest and abdomen compression, forcing air out and allowing the chest to expand and new air to flow in.

The Silvester Method was developed in 1858 by Henry Robert Silvester, a British physician interested in resuscitation and public health. This method was one of the earliest structured approaches to artificial respiration. The victim was placed on their back (supine) while the

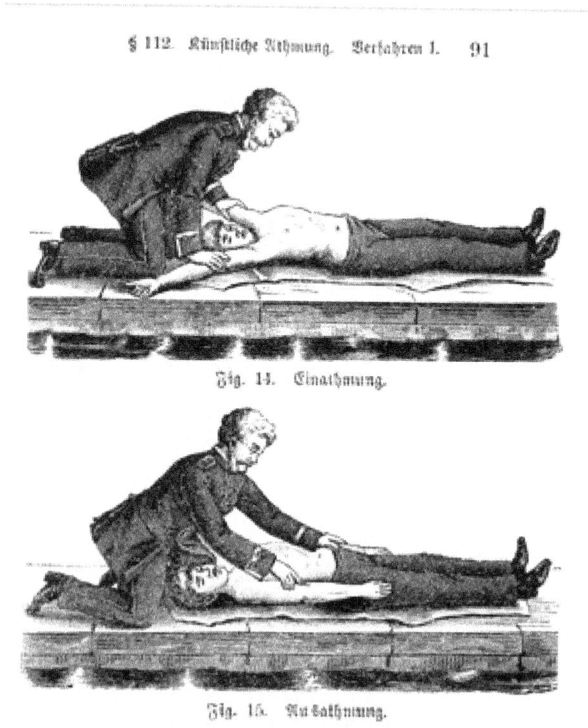

rescuer used rhythmic arm movements to stimulate breathing. The rescuer would raise the victim's arms over their head to expand the chest for inhalation, then press them down against the chest for exhalation. This technique introduced a repeatable, teachable process at a time when resuscitation was inconsistent and often improvised. This clearly demonstrated that mechanical chest movement could simulate breathing, and it brought structure, improved timing, and rhythm into lifesaving efforts. The Silvester Method was adopted by lifesaving societies as a standard approach, and it was widely used in drowning rescues, maritime settings, and in early first aid training. Although it established controlled, rhythmic artificial respiration, the amount of air exchange was limited and varied. The outcomes depended on precise execution, prompting the need for more efficient, effective ventilation methods.

Things could have taken quite a developmental leap in 1891, when German doctor Friedrich Maass performed the first closed-chest cardiac massage in a human. At that time, extensive surgery was required to perform cardiac massage, so using just pressure was a huge deal. Maass published his findings in German, and perhaps the medical world wasn't ready for his radically simple idea. Consequently, his contribution was largely ignored for decades, and the spark he struck wouldn't catch fire for half a century.

In 1903 in the United Kingdom, Sir Edward Albert Sharpey-Schafer developed the Schafer Method, which is also known as the "prone pressure method." The victim is placed face down with their head turned to the side to keep the airway open. The rescuer kneels over the victim's hips and firmly presses on the flank, compressing the abdomen for two to three seconds. This is repeated about 12 times per minute.

The pressure forces air out of the lungs (exhalation), and when released, the chest naturally expands, allowing air to flow back in (inhalation), thus simulating breathing.

This method improved upon earlier techniques by using body weight instead of arm movements, making it more practical and effective. It also reinforced the importance of consistent rhythm and positioning in resuscitation. This method was also easier to teach. The Schafer Method was widely adopted by organizations such as the Red Cross, Boy Scouts, and British Army.

Together, the Silvester Method and the Schafer Method transformed resuscitation from improvised efforts into systematic, teachable procedures centered on positioning, rhythm, and controlled mechanical ventilation. They represent a critical progression in the early development of artificial respiration. Silvester introduced a structured, rhythmic technique using arm movements to expand and compress the chest, establishing that breathing could be mechanically simulated in a repeatable way. Schafer advanced this concept by shifting to a prone position and using direct pressure on the back, improving practicality and reinforcing the use of body weight and consistent pressure cycles.

However, neither approach produced adequate, consistent air exchange. Plus, they both required precise execution to be effective. These challenges highlighted the need for a method that could better coordinate movement, pressure, and ventilation efficiency.

In 1932, Holger Nielsen, a military drill sergeant and gymnastics instructor in Denmark, would combine concepts from the Silvester Method and the Schafer Method into one system, the Hogler Nielsen Technique.

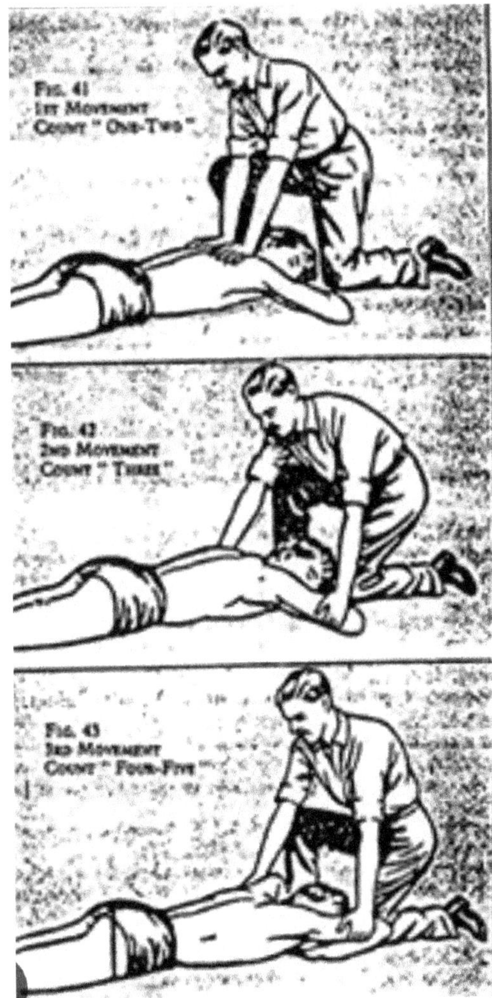

If you're like me, after reading that Nielsen was a drill sergeant and gymnastics instructor, you are conjuring up images of military personnel doing acrobatics or stunts on the parallel bars, but at that time, gymnastics instructors were more like military fitness trainers. Nielsen trained soldiers, police officers, firefighters, and lifeguards in the importance of body mechanics, movement control, symmetry, posture correction, and fitness—based on his Nordic culture and training. Body mechanics focused on using the body efficiently while carrying a load, which was training he provided for firefighters and the military. There was an emphasis on proper lifting, weight distribution and avoidance of fatigue and injury.

Movement control stressed deliberate coordinated movement patterns that were smooth and controlled versus forceful or erratic. Participants practiced maintaining muscle control during exertion. Examples of movement control are controlled lifting and lowering and coordinated team movements like stretcher handling. They did repetitive drills to standardize motion. Symmetry trains the body to work evenly and balanced to avoid twisting or uneven strain and over-reliance on one side.

These practices improve endurance, reduce injury, and maintain efficiency. They encouraged soldiers to observe controlled positioning of their spine, arms, and legs to better manage stability during stress. This improved efficiency while moving in sync when carrying or lifting.

In Nielsen's time (the late 19th to the early 20th century), the Physical Culture Movement was a big, big deal. It was a widespread effort across Sweden, Germany, the United Kingdom, and the United States to improve health, strength, and discipline through structured exercise. The Physical Culture Movement emphasized controlled movement, symmetry, posture, and breathing, using systems like calisthenics and gymnastics rather than competitive sport. These concepts were adopted in schools, the military, and public programs. This train of thought treated the body as something to be trained deliberately and efficiently, linking physical fitness to personal responsibility and societal strength. Scandinavian countries contended that strong, disciplined bodies equated to a strong, disciplined nation. Men and boys of that era were trained in breathing exercises, calisthenics, posture correction, lifesaving techniques (including swimming), proper hygiene, and public health principles.

Other factors that might have contributed to the popularity of the movement include people moving into the cities and away from farming and physical labor. Some idealists wanted to ensure that their military enlistees were well nourished prior to joining the military. Health enthusiasts pushed for more physical activity to improve health.

Nielsen drew these conclusions from his extensive empirical knowledge of chest expansion mechanics, posture, and respiration, combined with his experience with controlled movement for physiological effect. This progression led to the development of the Nielsen method, which built directly on the foundations of Silvester and Schafer, by refining body positioning and synchronized mechanical movements, representing the next step in the evolution of artificial respiration.

In the Hogler Nielsen Technique, the rescuer kneels at the victim's head. The non-responsive person is placed in a prone position, and their head is turned to one side to help keep the airway open. The rescuer places both hands on the victim's back, just below the shoulder blades, and leans forward, applying firm downward pressure. This compresses the chest and forces air out of the lungs. This is the exhalation or pressure phase. The inhalation phase commences when the rescuer releases the pressure, then grasps their arms near the elbows and lifts them up and out. This expands the chest and allows air to flow into the lungs. This cycle is repeated rhythmically about 10 to 12 times per minute. This was the most effective manual breathing simulation—until modern CPR.

Chapter 2: Where the Sparks Ignited

Scan to learn more about CPR history.

Finally, after about 75 more years, the sparks of the CPR movement began to catch! It seems only right that this happened in the heart of it all—the great state of Ohio, in the city of Cleveland.

In 1947, cardiac surgeon Dr. Claude S. Beck performed the first successful human defibrillation during open heart surgery on a 14-year-old boy named Richard Heyard at Case Western Reserve University. Defibrillation is the delivery of a controlled electrical shock to the heart to stop a life-threatening abnormal rhythm.

The most common arrhythmias are ventricular fibrillation (VF) or pulseless ventricular tachycardia (VT). The shock allows the heart's normal rhythm to resume. VF typically occurs when the heart becomes electrically unstable, most often during a heart attack or due to an underlying heart condition. During VF, the heart is not "stopped." It is electrically active but mechanically ineffective, quivering instead of pumping and unable to circulate blood.

Dr. Beck's first successful human defibrillation was not performed in a controlled lab test. It was during a real emergency, on a real human boy! During surgery to correct pectus excavatum, a sunken chest, Richard's heart went into VF. His heart was not circulating blood and oxygen throughout his body. Dr. Beck manually massaged Richard's heart for 45 minutes, then he used his defibrillator to shock it and initiate the return of spontaneous circulation.

Dr. Beck proved something many doctors still doubted: A heart rhythm *can* be restored.

You might be wondering how Dr. Beck had a defibrillator, which were uncommon back then. In 1947, defibrillators were limited to a very small number of researchers and surgeons working in experimental settings.

> The first successful human defibrillation was not performed in a controlled lab test. It was during a real emergency, on a real human boy!

Apparently, Dr. Beck was inspired by his colleague Carl J. Wiggers, a physiologist who had successfully restarted the hearts of lab animals with electrical shocks. Dr. Beck designed a defibrillator, and it was built by his friend James Rand III.

Remember when I said that I thought that CPR was born out of desperation? Dr. Beck was scared by the death of a young boy in the 1930s, whose heart began to fibrillate during surgery. Dr. Beck later stated that his inability to save the child burned a hole in his heart. I imagine that when the opportunity to try even his experimental device to save young Richard, he ordered his staff to retrieve his device and bring it to the operating room.

During Richard's recovery, he was said to be anxious to get back to his studies, given his second chance at life. As he grew into adulthood, he was an icon of successful defibrillation, and he even gave public appearances. Later, he worked as a machinist, and he married and had a son, who grew up to become a science teacher and often cited his father's medical advancement miracle as the reason his family had the opportunity to be created.

Dr. Beck's work laid the foundation for future defibrillation and CPR techniques. As not to be confusing, we will take a more in-depth look at defibrillation as a development in chapter 3. Dr. Beck and his colleagues didn't stop with the successful defibrillation of Richard Heyard. Throughout the 1940s and 1950s, they developed early cardiac rescue protocols. Their message was clear: Cardiac arrest didn't have to mean death if you moved fast enough.

The ripple effect of that message was real, moving from Ohio operating rooms to national medical journals. Ohio's early leadership in cardiac care helped shape modern CPR and AED developments worldwide. That mindset forged in Ohio laid the groundwork for modern resuscitation. Without the breakthroughs in Cleveland, lifesaving tools like CPR and defibrillators would have been delayed by years.

In 1954, Dr. James Otis Elam, an anesthesiologist and US military physician working at Roswell Park Memorial Institute in Buffalo, New York, conducted experiments on people who volunteered to be pharmacologically paralyzed so that they wouldn't be able to breathe. To me, it's remarkable that anyone would volunteer for that, but Dr. Elam's data proved that positive pressure ventilation (mouth-to-mouth) was an effective substitution for breathing for another person. It also showed that mouth-to-mouth was superior to previous methods, such as the Bellows Method and the Holger Nielsen Method, in laboratory settings. This showed that people's expired air is not "waste gas," which was a popular notion of the time.

Dr. Elam's first findings were published in military and medical research settings. Then in the late 1950s, they were formalized into peer-reviewed journals, including the *Journal of the American Medical Association* and the *Archives of Internal Medicine.*

Dr. Elam became painfully aware that what healthcare practitioners were doing to ventilate patients, including the Holger Nielsen Technique, was not good enough. He knew that patients were not getting enough oxygen, although he didn't yet have the data to prove it. He conducted clinical research and proved that if a person was not breathing, someone else could breathe for them. Dr. Elam developed a prototype ventilator that could effectively absorb carbon dioxide during surgery. This evolved into the Air-Shields Ventimeter ventilator, an early automatic respirator and neonatal ventilator that was used for about 50 years.

Dr. Elam's birth and early career offer insights into why he might have conducted the research that he did. According to the book *Human Progress, Science Heroes* and some professional anesthesiology journals, James Elam was born prematurely and weighed only two pounds at birth. Allegedly, the doctor told his mother that if he stopped breathing, she should stimulate him by rubbing or tapping him. Elam might have had breathing problems growing up, which might have influenced some of his career choices. He definitely was interested in respiratory science and went on for advanced physiology training at the University of Minnesota.

Early in Dr. Elam's career, he treated many patients with polio, some of whom were paralyzed and unable to breathe. They used a ventilator commonly called the iron lung, but when there were not enough machines to go around, Dr. Elam ventilated patients by mouth-to-mouth, although that was considered to be unhygienic and frowned upon at that time, and it had not yet become common medical practice. Instead, doctors still preferred to use bellow devices with ventilation bags, the Schafer Method, and the Holger Nielsen Technique.

Later, Dr. Elam partnered with Dr. Peter Safar to promote rescue breathing, the idea of breathing for someone else, as a viable lifesaving technique. Of the two men, Dr. Safar is more commonly known, having been the more public-facing partner. But perhaps Dr. Elam should be acknowledged as the Father of Resuscitation, if we are giving out titles and such. More on Dr. Safar coming up.

Around the same time, in 1956 in Boston, inspired by Dr. Beck's work, Dr. Paul M. Zoll developed and demonstrated external closed chest defibrillation. Now lethal heart dysrhythmia could be treated without opening the chest cavity. By that time, Dr. Zoll had already created the first external pacemaker that used electrical impulses via chest electrodes placed on the chest. That external pacemaker was the ancestor to transcutaneous pacing and implanted pacemakers.

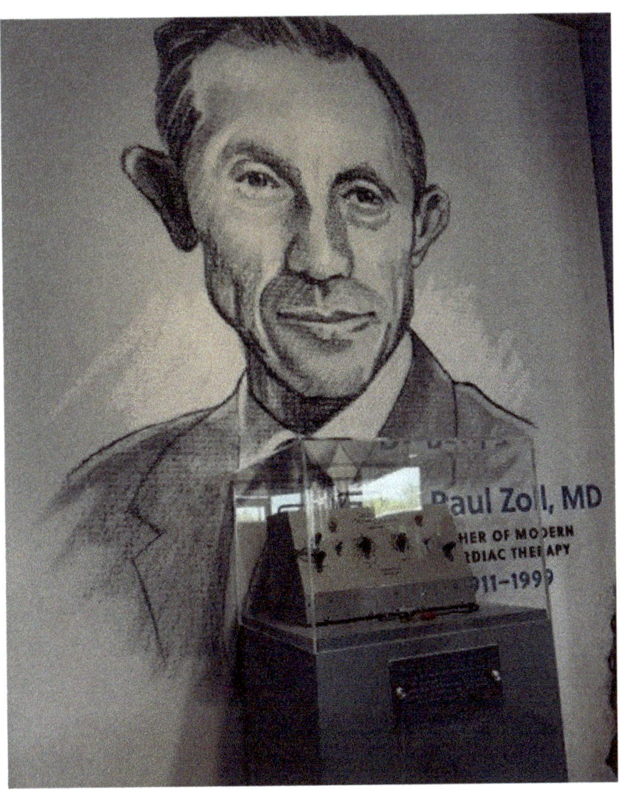

Dr. Zoll was born in 1911 in Boston to Hyman and Mollie Homsky Zoll, Eastern European Jewish immigrants from the Lithuania/Belarus region. He was one of two sons. It is highly likely that Hyman worked in the leather or garment trade business, and Mollie was reported to have had a home electrolysis business, which was a popular beauty service home business at that time. When Mollie was just 49 years old, she passed away—either due to cardiac insufficiency or rheumatic heart disease. That was during Dr. Zoll's final year at medical school, and it could be why he chose to carry on her love of electricity. But instead of using electricity to beautify, Dr. Zoll used it to save lives.

Before Mollie died, she requested that an autopsy be performed on her body to help doctors learn and to help more people. That created a major rift in the family because Dr. Zoll supported her wishes, but his father, Hyman, did not, due to his religious beliefs.

Mollie's passing might have fueled Dr. Zoll's obsession with solving the electrical failures of the heart. He became a cardiologist innovator and served as a US Army physician during World War II and as Chief of the Cardiac Clinic at Beth Israel Hospital from 1947 through 1958.

Because of Dr. Zoll, we are able to use defibrillators in the hospital and beyond. In 1980, the ZOLL Medical Corporation was founded in his honor, which has maintained leadership in AEDs and cardiac monitors. To this day, Dr. Zoll's innovations remain central to emergency cardiovascular care.

In 1956, it all started to come together. Let's get back to Dr. Peter Safar, a dynamic Vienna, Austria-born physician who was formally trained as an anesthesiologist. He immigrated to the United States, and he mainly lived in Pittsburgh, Pennsylvania. He worked with Dr. Elam to expound upon his work and initiate a system refining airway techniques, such as the head-tilt chin lift.

As the story goes, after Dr. Elam and Dr. Safar attended a Society of Anesthesiologist dinner in Kansas, Dr. Elam asked to hitch a ride back to Baltimore with Dr. Safar. This gave the two plenty of time to discuss anything! That is like a 16- to 18-hour drive. The anesthesiologists chose to debate the pros and cons of various resuscitative methods.

Dr. Elam explained that he had proven that exhaled air was adequate for rescue breaths. At the time, many physicians believed that exhaled air was "used up" and contained little to no usable oxygen, making it unsuitable for resuscitation. Dr. Elam challenged that assumption, demonstrating that exhaled breath still contained enough oxygen to support life. He saw a clear contradiction between what worked in controlled settings and what was being done in emergencies, and he set out to fix it, asking, "If direct ventilation works in the operating room, why aren't we using it everywhere?" Although Dr. Elam proved scientifically that mouth-to-mouth resuscitation was superior to the Holger Nielsen Technique and other techniques, mouth-to-mouth had not been widely accepted and was viewed as unhygienic. His work was convincing, but limited in scale.

Then Dr. Safar suggested that exhaled air from mouth-to-mouth breathing provides sufficient oxygen to a non-breathing person. Later, he conducted a series of experiments proving it. They concluded that they should collaborate. Dr. Elam had proven that rescue breaths were more efficient and consistent at providing ventilation. Dr. Safar designed the experiments that helped garner the data needed to solidify that this technique was efficient and repeatable. Dr. Safar took Dr. Elam's findings, standardized the method and tested it systematically, and directly compared it to the Holger Nielsen Technique.

The two physicians went on to establish the initial steps of CPR, including the head-tilt maneuver to open the patient's airway, and the exact method and positioning of mouth-to-mouth rescue breathing. In 1957, Dr. Safar published the book *The ABCs of Resuscitation*, introducing the Airway, Breathing, Circulation Method, which became the basis for CPR training. The ABC sequence would last as science for at least 50 years.

In 1958, Dr. Safar and Dr. Elam coauthored pivotal studies that showed rescue breathing and chest compressions together had the power to bring people back from clinical death. Their work was published in the *New England Journal of Medicine*.

Dr. Safar didn't stop there. He saw gaps in emergency care: People were dying before help arrived. He taught CPR to firefighters, and he helped create the first emergency medicine systems. He collaborated with national and international medical organizations, including the American Heart Association, to create training protocols and global CPR standards. Emergency medicine and resuscitation science programs were founded based on these developments, creating the backbone of modern CPR.

He believed that lifesaving skills belonged to the public, not just doctors and medical professionals. Because of Dr. Safar, CPR had a champion—and a pulse. He's often called the Father of CPR.

In 1960, American electrical engineer William Bennet Kouwenhoven published a groundbreaking paper introducing the breaths and chest compression CPR that we use today. Kouwenhoven had discovered the value of external cardiac compression by accident. A dog was in cardiac arrest, and heavy paddles had been placed on its chest. The weight increased the dog's blood pressure. Kouwenhoven realized that rhythmic pressure on the dog's sternum could maintain adequate circulation to the brain.

Today, the American Red Cross calls Kouwenhoven the Father of Modern CPR. He famously said, "Anyone can initiate cardiac resuscitation procedures anywhere. All that is needed are two hands."

"Anyone can initiate cardiac resuscitation procedures anywhere. All that is needed are two hands."
—William Bennet Kouwenhoven, the Father of Modern CPR

By 1960, we can see the rhythm forming, the Pulse Behind the Push. At the Johns Hopkins University in Baltimore, Maryland, three gentleman I like to call the John Hopkins Trio, William Kouwenhoven, an electrical engineer and professor of engineering; Dr. James Jude, a cardiac surgeon; and Dr. Guy Knickerbocker, a doctoral student and electrical researcher. That groundbreaking team showed that forceful, rhythmic external chest compressions could circulate blood effectively without opening up the chest, such as during cardiac arrest. They were inspired by the earlier work of Dr. Claude Beck and his successful defibrillation. The trio's published findings cemented CPR as a viable, worthwhile structured emergency response procedure.

This method changed the C in the CPR ABC formula from *circulation* to *compression*. Chest compressions added to Dr. Safar and Dr. Elam's rescue breathing equaled true cardiopulmonary resuscitation.

The trio published groundbreaking research showing that external chest compressions could revive cardiac arrest victims without surgery. That was the first time a noninvasive method was shown to restore circulation and prevent brain death. Their work turned the idea of emergency response into a physical action that anyone could do. This advancement led to the modern integration of compressions in CPR protocols. Their work gave people the power to keep a heart pumping until help arrives, saving millions of lives.

The 1950s and 1960s were a buzzing time for CPR development, and a lot of things were happening within a short proximity of each other. Before we get ahead of ourselves, it is difficult to *teach* CPR if there is no victim or manikin! In order to teach, you need tools. Back then, there were no manikins, so Dr. Elam and Dr. Safar approached Norwegian toy maker Asmund Laerdal with a bold request: to create the first realistic CPR training manikin to teach people how to save lives.

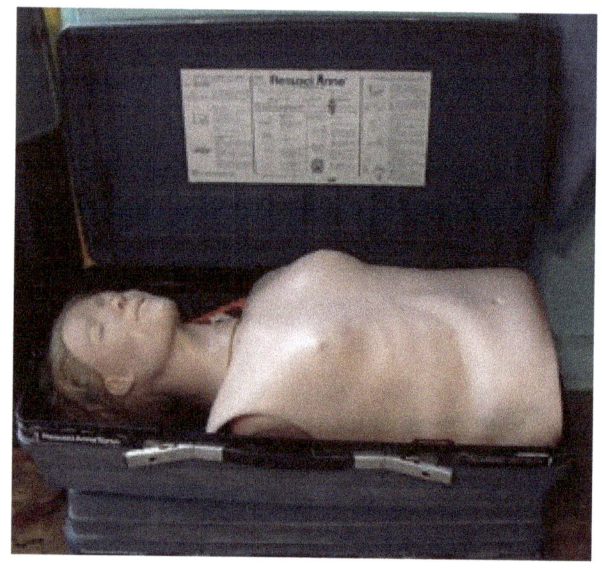

Laerdal created the first CPR training manikin, released in 1960, which was later named Resusci Anne. The training manikin had a human-like face based on the death mask of a drowned girl. This manikin enabled CPR to be teachable to the masses. Originally, the manikin was called "Resuscitation Anne," but the name was shortened for ease of international reference. In the United States, we often call her Rescue Annie.

You might be wondering, *Is it manikin or mannequin?* Mannequins are stationary, full-bodied models used in retail to display clothing. Manikins are specialized, often anatomically correct, models used for medical training, CPR, or scientific purposes.

To create Resusci Anne, Laerdal used soft vinyl skin that had been originally intended for toy dolls, real anatomical landmarks like the nipple line and the xiphoid process, and an airway system so people could properly practice mouth-to-mouth breathing and chest compressions. Laerdal modeled the face after a mysterious drowned girl whose body was pulled from the Seine in the 1880s, *L'Inconnue de la Seine*. Her serene-looking death mask had become a symbol of lost potential and quiet beauty. Laerdal believed that her peaceful expression would make people more comfortable practicing lifesaving skills. It's ironic that the face of a girl who was not saved from drowning became the tool that taught the world how to save others. Her image became the global standard training tool for CPR.

Interesting, right? Death masks were common during that era because they captured the last expression of a person. Photographs weren't common yet. Death masks were used to record, identify, study, and remember a person's face at the moment of death. They preserved the likeness of a person. It was common for well-known, famous people to have death masks made, usually in their homes or by memorial personnel. Death masks were not usually created for regular folks. However, they were sometimes created in morgues.

In late-19th-century Paris, the boundaries between medicine, public life, and art were more fluid than they are today. Paris was both academically grounded and experimentally driven, and formal institutions like the *École des Beaux-Arts* existed alongside independent, boundary-pushing artists. At that time in Paris, unidentified missing persons were displayed for the public, with their bodies preserved behind glass with their personal effects at the Paris Morgue. Even places like the Paris Morgue became part of the city's curiosity and cultural experience. As a vibrant cultural hub, Paris brought together writers, philosophers, scientists, and artists, allowing ideas to move quickly across disciplines.

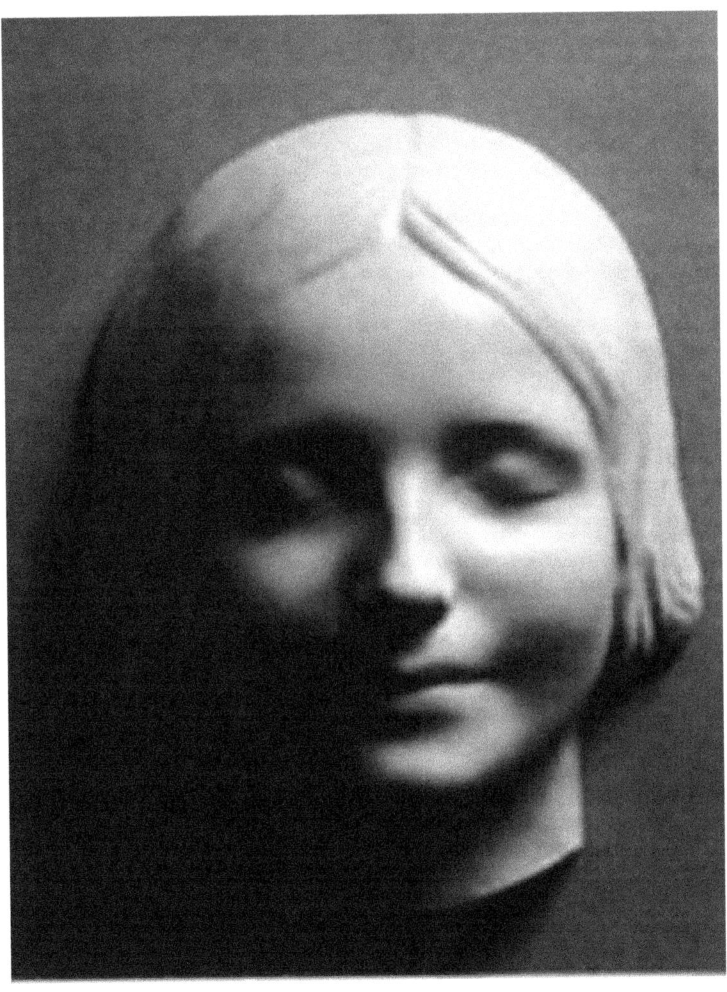

In late-19th-century Paris, medicine, public spectacle, and art intersected, and an unidentified woman's face might have been cast for official purposes or through individual curiosity or aesthetic interest. Once the drowned girl's death mask was introduced into Paris' artistic network, the mask was reproduced and circulated, transforming it from an anonymous death mask into a widely shared cultural object.

I believe that Laerdal was predestined—or at the very least inspired—to create the first CPR manikin. In 1954, he was forever changed when his young son, Tore Laerdal, nearly drowned. Laerdal saved his son with rescue breathing. That experience gave Laerdal a personal understanding of the terror of an emergency and the power of quick action. He believed in accessible education, and he wanted *everyone,* not just medical professionals, to have the training and confidence to step in and save a life. With his manikin, Laerdal made CPR training hands-on and accessible. He turned the *theory* of being able to teach CPR into a *reality.*

As I mentioned earlier, the 1960s was quite the vibe for CPR creation and advancement. And desperation still fueled the need for CPR. Sadly, in 1966, Dr. Safar's 11-year-old daughter, Elisabeth, suffered a severe asthma attack and prolonged oxygen deprivation. After her death, Dr. Safar's mission became personal. The loss fueled his mission, and he poured his pain into building better emergency response systems focused on preserving brain function. He hoped to save other parents from suffering in helplessness in a life-threatening situation.

The 1960s and 1970s brought a lot of scientific advancement. The American Heart Association (AHA), the American Red Cross, the National Academy of Sciences, and other organizations endorsed CPR. Also, the American Red Cross began funding CPR research.

AMERICAN HEART ASSOCIATION
CARDIOPULMONARY RESUSCITATION AND EMERGENCY CARDIAC CARE

PERFORMANCE TEST FOR UNWITNESSED CARDIAC ARREST ONE & TWO RESCUERS

NAME: ______ SS#: ______ DATE: ______

ELAPSED TIME (Seconds) Min.	Max.	ACTIVITY AND TIME (Seconds)	CRITICAL PERFORMANCE	PASS	FAIL
6	10	Establish unresponsiveness. Allow 4-10 sec. if face down and turning is required.	Shake shoulder, Shout - "Are you OK?" Turn if necessary. Adequate time		
7	15	Open airway Establish breathlessness (3 - 5 sec.)	Kneels properly Right hand under neck, left on forehead Ear over mouth		
10	20	Four Ventilations (3 - 5 sec.)	Ventilate 4 times [illegible] Adequate time		
15	30	Establish pulselessness (5 - 10 sec.)	Right hand palpates properly Adequate time		
75	95	Four cycles of 15 Compressions 2 Ventilations (60-65 sec.)	Proper body position Landmark check Position of hands Vertical compression [illegible] Proper rate Proper ratio No bouncing Ventilates adequately		
10	100	Establish return of pulse and spontaneous breathing & evaluate pupil (5 sec.)	Check pulse, breathing and pupil		
80	100	Minimum of two cycles of 5 Compressions-1 Ventilation. Switch & repeat until examiner is satisfied	Changes rate of compression [illegible] Interposes breath No pause for ventilation Calls for switch Switches Switches back Checks pulse (by ventilator) Checks pupil (by ventilator) Technique as above		

For single rescuer - Number of Compressions 60 ____ Number of Ventilations 12
Single rescue technique (check) Pass____ Fail____
Two person rescue technique Pass____ Fail____

Instructor: ______ (check) Pass____ Fail____

It's safe to say that developments in cardiac science in general led to developments in CPR science as well. The AHA had been focused on all things cardiac since the 1920s. In fact, since 1949, the AHA has invested more than $5 *billion* in cardiovascular and stroke research. By 1966, the AHA began helping to present national CPR conferences. By the 1970s, the AHA developed standardized Basic Life Support (BLS) and Advanced Cardiac Life Support (ACLS) courses.

Let's rewind a bit. A precursor to the AHA was founded in 1915 when a group of physicians and social workers in New York convened to uncover the mysteries of heart disease. They called their new organization the Association for the Prevention and Relief of Heart Disease. Not quite as catchy as the American Heart Association, right? One of the founding members, Dr. Paul Dudley White, stated that it was to combat the "unbelievable ignorance and poor prognosis surrounding heart disease." Its aim was to coordinate, research, and improve clinical care conditions by educating physicians. The cardiologists were primarily concerned with rheumatic heart disease and cardiovascular conditions of the era.

In 1924, the organization formally adopted the name the American Heart Association. It was officially founded in 1924 in Chicago by six physicians—Dr. Paul Dudley White, Dr. Lewis A. Conner, Dr. Robert H. Halsey, Dr. James B. Herrick, Dr. Hugh McCulloch, and Dr. Joseph Sailer—as a scientific professional medical society for doctors. This change reflected a broader, national focus on cardiovascular disease—rather than narrower clinical concerns.

In 1948, the AHA underwent a major reorganization, transforming from a physician-led professional society into a professionally-led national health organization that was supported by a broad base of volunteers. This restructuring allowed for public membership, nationwide fundraising, and large-scale community education. The AHA had evolved to include far more than the education of physicians.

Today, the AHA is still composed of volunteers, led and supported by a professional staff. The AHA became a national leader in funding cardiovascular research in public health education and a key driver in public health campaigns for heart disease, stroke prevention, circulatory health, and CPR education. Their publishing of scientific findings helped institutionalize Good Samaritan protections, which are laws that protect people who provide emergency assistance from liability, as long as they act in good faith and within reasonable standards of care. Those standards were defined and reinforced through evidence-based guidelines and training.

The 1950s and 1960s saw a great expansion of the AHA's public health influence. At the First National Conference on Cardiopulmonary Resuscitation in 1966, the first techniques of CPR were standardized. The 1960s and 1970s were more of an emergency cardiac care era. As resuscitation science advanced, the AHA became increasingly involved in supporting CPR research, emergency cardiovascular care, and the dissemination of lifesaving practices to both healthcare professionals and the public. The AHA formally endorsed CPR training for the general public and accelerated nationwide CPR education programs and integration into schools, workplaces, and community organizations by 1974. The National Academy of Sciences-National Research Council convened in response to requests from the American Red Cross and other federal agencies of the time about CPR. This gathering united representatives from

30 national organizations to review evidence and contribute recommendations for guidelines, target audiences and collaboration. The AHA took a leadership role and became a dominant voice in emergency cardiovascular care.

Ever since, the AHA has been recognized as a global authority in cardiovascular and stroke science, emergency cardiovascular care, and evidence-based guideline development. The organization continues to issue regular CPR and related courses, updates every five years in collaboration with the International Liaison Committee on Resuscitation (ILCOR).

The AHA has evolved from a small professional association into one of the most influential public health organizations in the world, driving innovation, CPR education, and cardiovascular research globally. The AHA publishes a family of medical journals, including *Circulation.* Also major medical findings have been published in the *Journal of the American Medical Association (JAMA).*

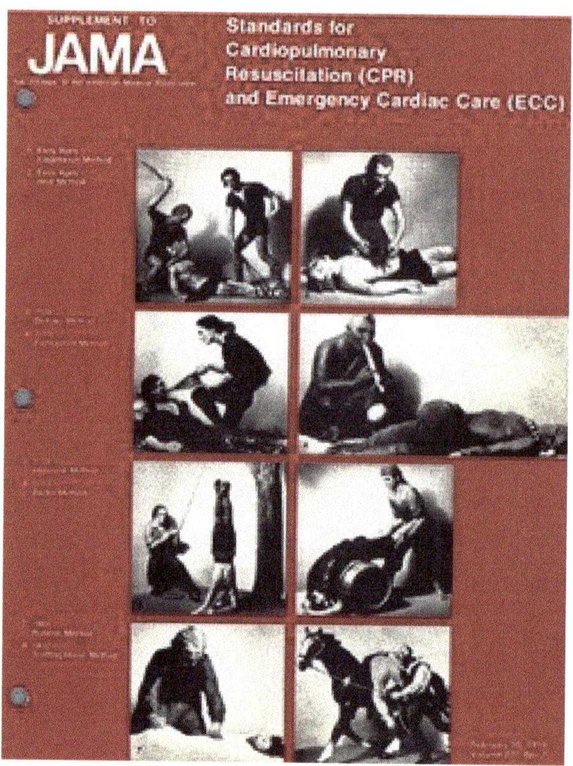

JAMA and the AHA journals often share research and collaborate to shape clinical practice and guidelines. *JAMA* was founded in 1883 to establish a platform to share medical research, clinical updates, and policy insights. It publishes cutting-edge biomedical research, reviews, and advocacy editorials. They are one of the most respected medical journals globally and a key player in shaping public health policies and ethical standards in medicine.

Together, the AHA and *JAMA* form the backbone of medical standardization in the United States. *JAMA* brought research and advocacy to the medical community, while the AHA brought CPR and cardiac care to the public. Together, they helped turn lifesaving science into standard global practice.

Chapter 3: Where the Beat Meets the Spark

Scan to learn more about CPR history.

Let's step back a moment and explore the development of Automated External Defibrillator (AED) development. It's easier to separate the paths of CPR and defibrillation development here to highlight AED evolution.

By the 1960s, the medical community knew that many adult occurrences of sudden cardiac arrest begin with ventricular fibrillation (VF) or pulseless ventricular tachycardia (VT). Therefore, the initial problem is not lack of oxygen but rather lack of *circulation*. The patient's heart's electrical system becomes chaotic, and the heart stops pumping effectively, disrupting blood flow to the heart and brain. Defibrillation delivers a shock (a therapeutic dose of electrical energy) to the heart to stop that chaotic electrical activity. This momentary electrical pause allows the heart's natural pacemaker to reset and resume a normal, organized rhythm.

That's why modern cardiac arrest treatment relies on the combined use of CPR and defibrillation. CPR maintains minimal circulation and supports the body until defibrillation can reset the heart's electrical rhythm.

The chest compressions of CPR generate partial circulation, typically producing about 20 to 30 percent of normal cardiac output and help maintain coronary perfusion pressure. This circulation helps deliver oxygen to the brain and heart and increases the likelihood that defibrillation will restore a normal rhythm.

Without CPR, VF can deteriorate into asystole, which is the complete absence of electrical activity in the heart. There is no heartbeat, no pulse, and no cardiac output. On a monitor, it appears as a flat—or nearly flat—line. Even when the heart stops pumping, oxygen remains in the blood for several minutes.

Defibrillation stop's the heart's chaotic electrical activity and resets the heart's electrical rhythm, but it does not *restart* the heart. The heart needs to use energy to recover and generate a normal rhythm. That's why defibrillation works better with CPR—when there is some oxygen and cellular energy reserve in the heart. An AED analyzes the heart's rhythm and delivers a shock when indicated.

CPR maintains minimal circulation and supports the body until defibrillation can reset the heart's electrical rhythm.

The discovery of defibrillation, the development of CPR, and the invention of AEDs combined to create our modern resuscitation systems. CPR provides temporary circulation, defibrillation restores electrical rhythm, and AEDs place lifesaving capability in the hands of the public. Together, they form the integrated survival model that underlies contemporary cardiac arrest treatment.

AEDs emerged from decades of research in electrophysiology, engineering, emergency medicine, and public health. There were a lot of people involved, and I am sure it was messy, especially because the sciences merged across countries, politics, education gaps, and resource shortages.

Long before scientists understood cardiac rhythm disturbances, investigators in the late 18th century began exploring the effects of electricity on living tissue.

Those early studies laid the scientific groundwork for later discoveries about the electrical nature of the heart. An early influential pioneer was Luigi Galvani (1737–1798), an Italian physician and anatomist at the University of Bologna. Dr. Galvani demonstrated through experiments with frogs' legs that electrical stimulation could cause muscles to contract. He hypothesized that living organisms contained an internal electrical force, which he termed "animal electricity." His work established the principle that electricity could directly influence biological tissues.

Other researchers were inspired by Dr. Galvani's work to explore potential medical uses of electricity. In 1788, English physician Charles Kite proposed using electrical stimulation as part of efforts to revive drowning victims. Around the same time, Giovanni Aldini, Galvani's nephew, was interested in "animal electricity," which was soon referred to as "Galvanism," and conducted public demonstrations showing that electrical currents could stimulate muscles in recently deceased bodies. Aldini traveled across Europe showing that electrical currents could stimulate muscles in dead animals and human bodies.

Who attended these events and where were they held? Times were different, and there were a lot of different opportunities and priorities. These events were attended by people in the medical community interested in the emerging science of electricity and physiology, natural philosophers, aka scientists, medical students, and the general public when permitted. They were held in medical schools and anatomical theaters, scientific societies, hospitals, medical lecture halls, and prisons immediately following executions. I guess these were educational regularities back then.

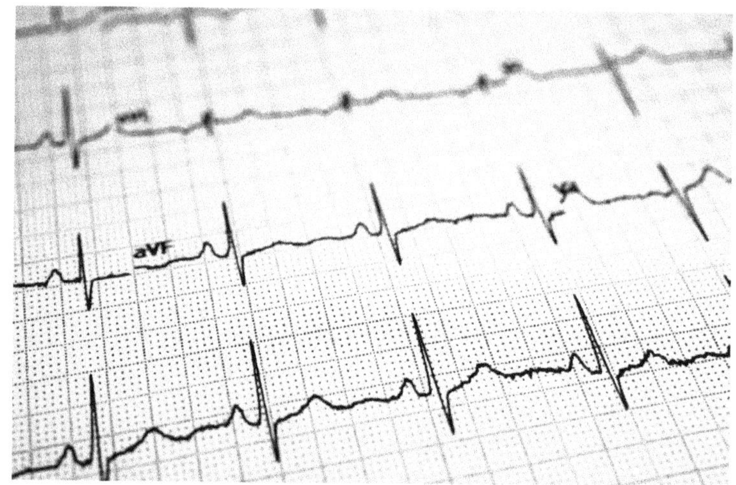

One famous demonstration occurred in London in 1803, when Aldini applied electrical stimulation to the body of George Forster, who had been executed at Newgate Prison, a notorious London jail. When electrical current was applied to Forster's face and limbs, the muscles contracted, causing movements of the jaw, eyes, and arms. Onlookers reported that the body appeared to move in lifelike ways, which generated substantial public interest and controversy. The demonstration was both scientifically intriguing and deeply unsettling for many observers. It was obvious these experiments did not restore life; however, they provided compelling evidence that electricity *could* activate muscles and nerves.

At the end of 19th century, two researchers at the University of Geneva demonstrated that electrical shocks could not only interrupt the heart's rhythm, but could also restore it.

These advancements reinforced the concept that electrical forces played a role in biological activity and contributed to early scientific discussions about the relationship between electricity and living tissue. These foundational concepts would later prove crucial and inspirational as scientists began investigating the possibility that electricity could be used to correct lethal cardiac rhythms.

Together, these early investigations helped establish the emerging field of bioelectricity and introduced the idea that electrical forces could influence bodily function. Previous investigations into bioelectricity demonstrated that electricity could stimulate muscles and nerves, but the correlation between electricity and the heart remained poorly understood. Throughout the 19th century, scientists continued researching how electrical currents affected cardiac tissue. At the end of the century, two researchers at the University of Geneva demonstrated that electrical shocks could not only interrupt the heart's rhythm, but could also restore it.

In 1899, Swiss physiologists Jean-Louis Prévost and Frédéric Batelli conducted a series of experiments that marked a turning point in the study of cardiac electrophysiology. Working with animal models, they demonstrated that electrical shocks could both *induce* ventricular fibrillation and *terminate* it. Their research established the principle that carefully applied electrical energy could restore normal cardiac rhythm, laying the foundation for the development of defibrillation therapy.

Despite this breakthrough, the concept of defibrillation did not immediately translate into clinical medical practice. Several obstacles slowed progress. At the time, physicians had limited understanding of cardiac electrophysiology and little ability to monitor heart rhythms during resuscitation attempts. Electrocardiography was still in its early stages, and the mechanisms of VF were not yet fully understood. Plus, electrical equipment capable of delivering controlled shocks to the heart had not yet been developed for medical use.

Asystole

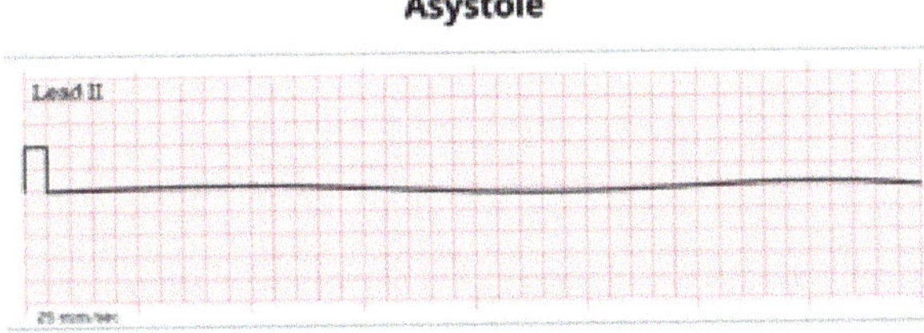

Throughout the early 20th century, researchers continued to investigate the electrical behavior of the heart in laboratory settings. Experimental physiologists studied cardiac rhythm disturbances and

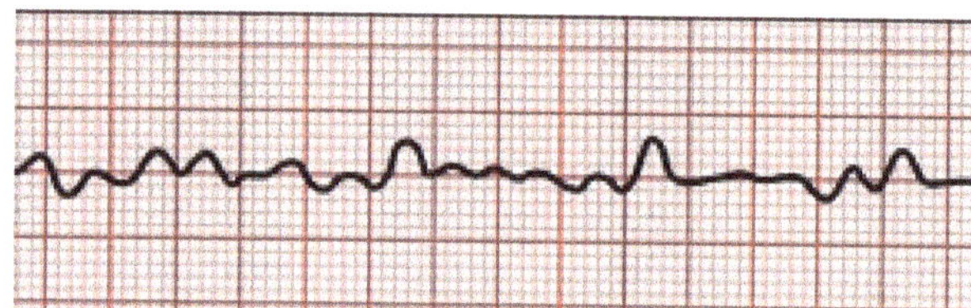

the effects of electrical stimulation on animal hearts, gradually expanding scientific knowledge about VF. The problem still remained, and practical clinical application remained elusive.

The period between 1899 and the 1940s represents a critical developmental stage in the history of defibrillation, a time when laboratory discoveries gradually evolved into practical medical therapy. During the early 20th century, several researchers continued studying the electrical behavior of the heart and the possibility of reversing lethal cardiac rhythms.

A major contributor was William Bennet Kouwenhoven, an electrical engineer at Johns Hopkins University. Beginning in the 1920s and 1930s, Kouwenhoven studied the effects of electrical currents on the human body, particularly in relation to electrical safety and accidental electrocution. His research helped determine how electrical shocks affect the heart, and it contributed to the development of safer defibrillation equipment. As previously mentioned, in 1960, Kouwenhoven played a central role in the discovery of modern closed-chest CPR.

Research on VF was also advanced by Dr. Harold S. Hyman, a cardiologist who explored electrical pacing and cardiac stimulation in the 1930s. Dr. Hyman developed an early artificial pacemaker intended to stimulate the heart using electrical impulses. Although his device was controversial at the time and not widely adopted, his work demonstrated that electrical technology *could* influence cardiac rhythm. It stimulated further interest in electrical therapies for the heart.

One of the most influential figures during this period was Carl J. Wiggers, an American physiologist in Cleveland, Ohio. Wiggers conducted extensive experimental studies on cardiac physiology and VF in the early 20th century. His laboratory work helped clarify how fibrillation develops and how electrical stimulation interacts with cardiac tissue. Wiggers's research provided much of the physiological understanding that later made clinical defibrillation possible.

The connection between Carl J. Wiggers and Claude Beck helps explain why the first successful human defibrillation occurred in Cleveland in 1947. Wiggers, a leading cardiovascular physiologist at Western Reserve University, spent decades studying the mechanics and electrical behavior of the heart. His laboratory became one of the most influential centers for cardiovascular research in the early 20th century. Wiggers and his colleagues conducted extensive experiments on VF, carefully documenting how the heart's rhythm deteriorates and how electrical stimulation affects cardiac tissue. Through those experiments, Wiggers helped establish a deeper understanding of the physiology of fibrillation and the conditions under which the heart might recover normal rhythm. His laboratory emphasized precise measurement of blood pressure, cardiac output, and electrical activity, producing detailed physiological data that shaped the emerging field of cardiac electrophysiology.

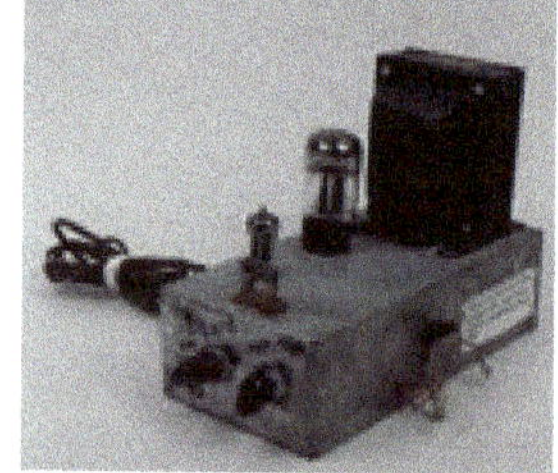

It was not until the 1930s and 1940s that surgeons began exploring the possibility of treating cardiac arrest directly during open-chest surgery. Remember Claude Beck? He operated in the same scientific environment influenced by Wiggers's work. Dr. Beck was interested in developing surgical methods to treat heart disease and became particularly concerned with the problem of sudden cardiac arrest during surgery. Drawing on the growing body of knowledge about VF and electrical stimulation, Dr. Beck began exploring whether direct electrical shocks could restore a normal rhythm when the heart entered fibrillation during an operation.

In 1947, Dr. Beck successfully terminated VF in a teenage patient during surgery by applying electrical paddles directly to the exposed heart. This event is widely recognized as the first successful human defibrillation. It confirmed that cardiac arrest could be treated with an open chest cavity. Dr. Beck's achievement demonstrated that the principles discovered decades earlier by Prévost and Batelli in laboratory experiments could indeed save a human life.

Together, Wiggers, Kouwenhoven, and Hyman built upon the early laboratory discoveries of Prévost and Batelli, paving the way for the clinical breakthroughs that would follow. Their research deepened scientific understanding of cardiac electrophysiology and contributed to the development of technologies capable of restoring normal heart rhythm.

Now that we have transitioned from laboratory science into clinical intervention, we can move on to the 1950s and 1960s. Dr. Paul Zoll demonstrated that electrical shocks could be delivered through the chest wall. He developed early external defibrillators, but they used alternating current, which could be unpredictable and cause myocardial injury. William Bennet Kouwenhoven, James Jude, and Guy Knickerbocker discovered closed chest cardiac massage in 1960, making resuscitation plausible without chest surgery. Dr. Bernard Lown, a Lithuanian-born American cardiologist, later introduced the direct current defibrillator, using capacitor discharge, which was shorter and controlled. Dr. Lown and engineers refined the technology into safer, more reliable devices. This intervention became safer for hospital use due to lower events of myocardial injury and more reliable rhythm conversion.

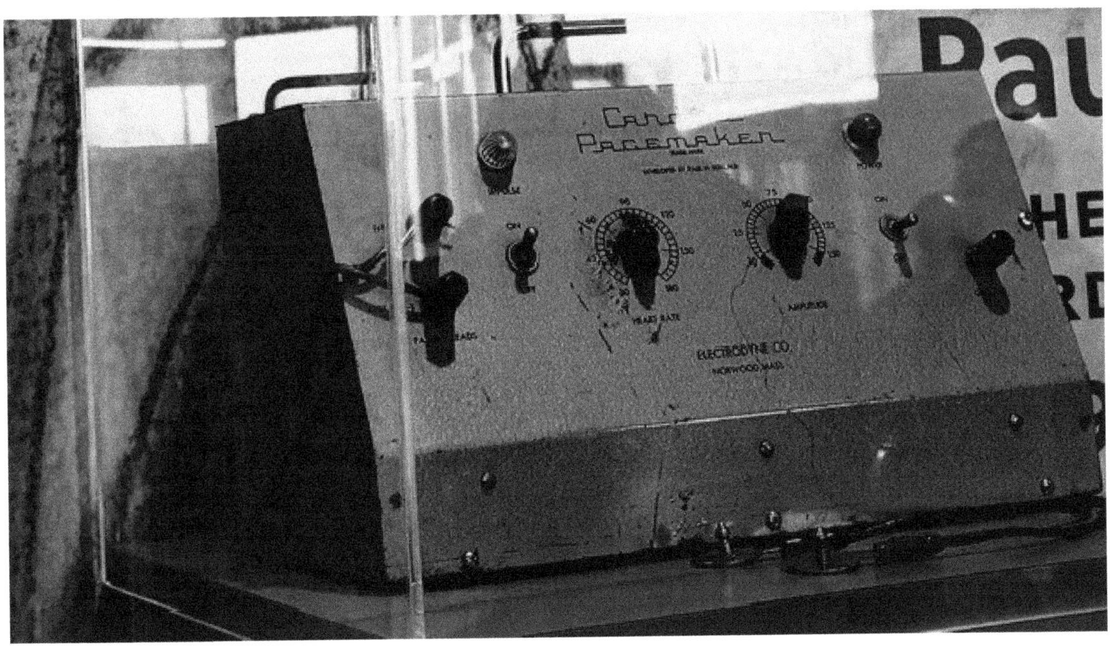

Portable defibrillators became possible when capacitor technology evolved dramatically during the aerospace era. Some early mobile defibrillator designs benefited from electronics developed for space missions. Dr. Arch Diack and his collaborators played a considerable role in developing early automated defibrillation systems that could analyze heart rhythms and guide rescuers. They were developing AEDs capable of detecting ventricular fibrillation (VF). These designs were mainly for paramedics and trained emergency personnel.

In 1972, former President Lyndon B. Johnson experienced a major heart attack while visiting his daughter in Charlottesville, Virginia. He was treated using a portable defibrillator, according to an article in *Smithsonian Magazine*. The device used was based on innovations by Irish cardiologist Frank Pantridge. He is often referred to as the Father of Emergency Medicine. His early designs evolved from a 150-pound, car battery-powered unit in 1965 to a significantly miniaturized version by the late 1960s, weighing approximately 7 pounds, made possible in part by capacitor technology developed for NASA. During President Johnson's emergency, a mobile coronary care unit (MCCU) from the University of Virginia Health System was dispatched, led by cardiologist Richard S. Crampton, delivering advanced cardiac care outside the traditional hospital setting.

President Johnson's high-profile case was an important public example of how emerging mobile cardiac care technologies could be used outside of traditional hospital settings. This case is widely credited with increasing public awareness of portable defibrillators and accelerating the adoption of mobile emergency cardiac care systems across the United States.

Modern defibrillators use biphasic waveforms that require less energy and produce better outcomes than earlier monophonic shocks. Biphasic technology became standard in most defibrillators in the late 1990s and early 2000s. This means biphasic shocks pass electrical current through the heart in two phases, which improves defibrillation success while requiring lower energy levels.

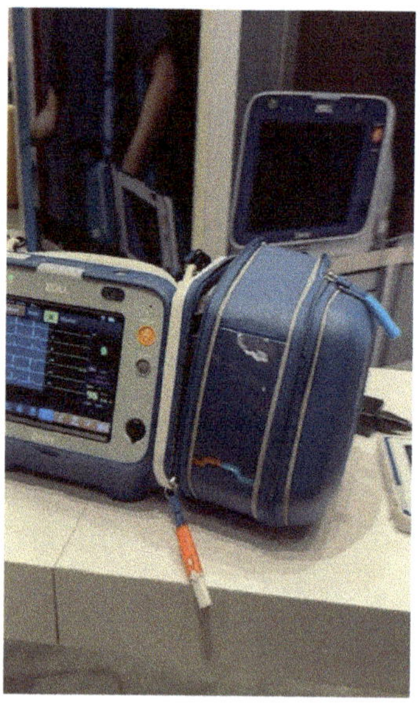

Mobile coronary care units, paramedic programs, and AED deployment brought defibrillation into public spaces. AEDs were then placed in public areas such as airports, arenas, casinos, malls, office buildings, and schools.

Research indicated that survival rates improve drastically when defibrillation occurs within three to five minutes of collapse. Published in 2000 in the *New England Journal of Medicine*, the Las Vegas Casino Study examined cardiac arrests occurring in several Las Vegas casinos where security staff were trained to use AEDs. The findings indicated that survival rates for witnessed VF cardiac arrest reached an estimated 53 percent. However, when defibrillation happened within three minutes, survival rates approached 74 percent. Rapid AED access significantly improved outcomes compared with historical survival rates.

During the 1980s and 90s, extreme advancements in microprocessors and batteries allowed AEDs to become small-

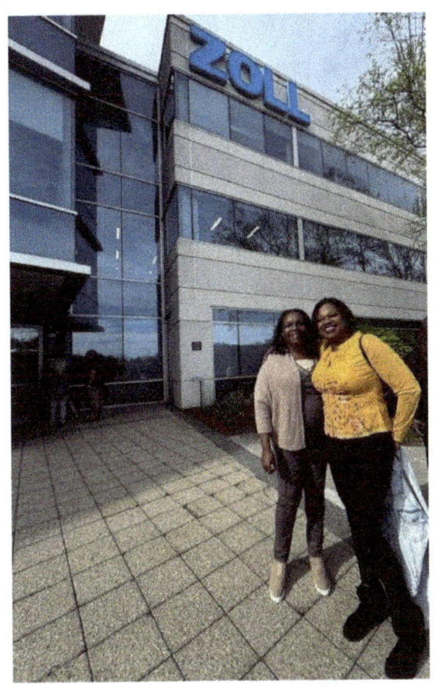

er and more user friendly. AEDs began to incorporate voice and visual prompts and automated rhythm detection. Today's AEDS are compact, widely distributed, and integrated with CPR feedback sensors, metronomes for compression rate guidance, real-time compression depth monitoring, and integration with emergency response systems. These features reinforce the partnership between CPR and defibrillation in modern cardiac arrest care.

Early major AED manufacturers include Medtronic, ZOLL, and Physio-Control. Today, the AED industry is led by a small group of global manufacturers—primarily Philips, ZOLL, and Stryker—alongside a network of international and emerging companies that expand access to defibrillation worldwide.

Avive is an emerging AED manufacturer bringing a new, connected approach to cardiac arrest response. Their connected AEDs integrate with emergency systems, providing real-time data, guidance, and improved accessibility—shifting AEDs from passive devices to active participants in cardiac arrest response.

Believe it or not, when AEDs were first introduced, they were controversial. There were legal battles over where AEDs should be placed. Businesses sometimes hesitated to install AEDs due to concerns that if the devices were improperly used, they would be responsible for someone's death. Initially, some states required physician oversight, formal training programs, EMS registration of devices, and maintenance protocols to use AEDs.

Over time, newer laws supported easier AED deployment. Today, many jurisdictions require AEDs in schools and institutions with many employees or attendees. Good Samaritan laws were implemented or expanded to encourage bystander AED use. These laws protect rescuers if they act in good faith, attempt emergency care, and follow basic guidelines.

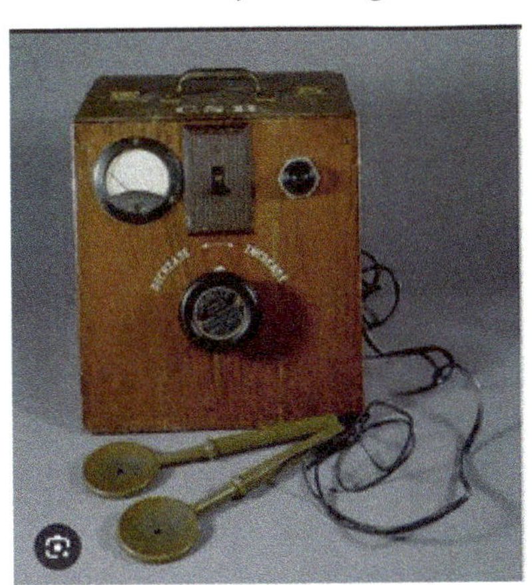

It's a good thing that we developed science and applicable guidelines that even specific industries adhere to. While editing this book, my neighbor—a retired military and civilian electrician—told me that his training manual in the 1970s said that to resuscitate an electrocuted person, you would grasp their tongue and stick your finger in their rectum! So even though my neighbor began training after CPR and AEDs had been created, not all of the information had filtered into all sectors and training manuals.

Upon researching this resuscitation method, I think they might have been trying to elicit the gasp response. I reckon that if someone did that to me, I would surely gasp if I could. I think I also would have gasped if I was the one to have to revive a crew member with that method, especially because wearing gloves wasn't common yet back then.

Around 2010, resuscitation guidelines replaced the ABC (airway, breathing, circulation) sequence with the CAB (compression, airway, breathing) sequence. This promotes faster initiation of chest compressions.

Research had shown that bystanders often hesitated or have difficulty with administering rescue breaths, and those delays reduced survival. Chest compressions create artificial circulation by increasing intrathoracic pressure and compressing the heart between the sternum and spine. Thus, beginning CPR with chest compressions shortens the time before compression commencement. This transition represents a deeper understanding of cardiac arrest physiology. Immediate circulation through chest compressions, combined with rapid defibrillation when needed, forms our current resuscitation practices.

It's amazing that it took all of that—and probably some other people and events—to get us to this point.

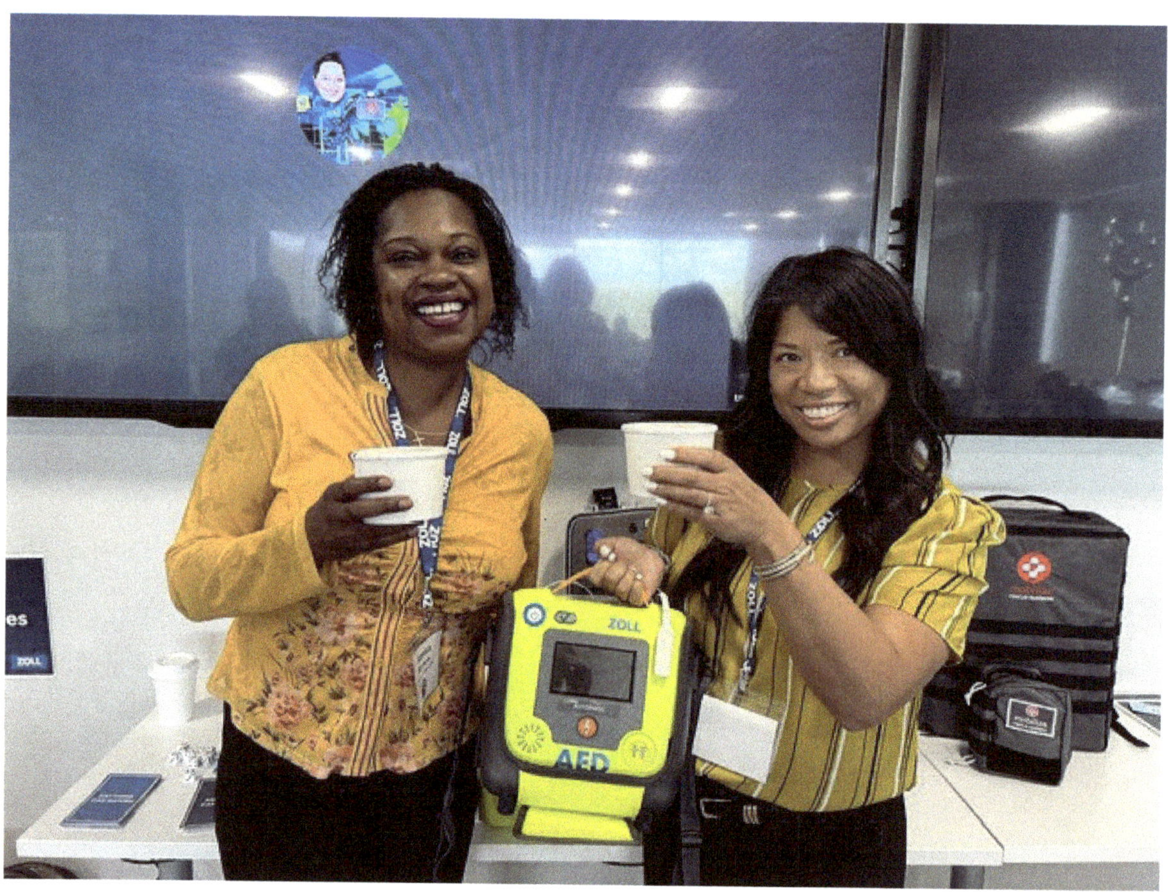

Chapter 4: The Birth of a Movement

Scan to learn more about CPR history.

Many forward-thinking experts, including Dr. Peter Safar and Dr. James Elam, advanced CPR science and got it out to the medical community. That was beneficial when a sudden cardiac event happened inside a hospital. However, *most* sudden cardiac arrests happen *outside* of hospital settings. Time is of the essence for getting those patients to a hospital.

We can all thank Dr. Leonard Cobb for realizing that CPR was not useful unless people *outside* of hospitals knew it and used it. He viewed cardiac arrest death as preventable. He believed that survival required community education, fast response, and citizen action.

It's pretty much because of Dr. Cobb that today public CPR training is the norm. Dr. Cobb is credited with bringing CPR out of the hospitals and into the communities. He knew that *everyone* could be a lifesaver. Personally, I would like to acknowledge all of the named and unnamed people who contributed to this venture. Yes, if we have to choose one person to get credit for bringing CPR to the masses, Leonard Cobb is that person, but the research, trials, exposure, funding, and inspiration came from *many* people.

Leonard Arthur Cobb was born on February 18, 1924, in Rochester, New York. His father was a physician who exposed young Leonard to early medical conversations, doctrine, and professional responsibility. He became aware of the realities of illness and mortality, clinical reasoning, and medical ethics. Leonard went on to study at Colgate University for his undergraduate degree, then at the University of Rochester School of Medicine, attaining his MD in 1949.

Dr. Cobb's internship and residency were in internal medicine, and he acquired specialized training in cardiology. He entered medicine during a time when heart disease was becoming the leading cause of death in America.

After medical school, Dr. Cobb served in the US Army Medical Corps. That experience exposed him to structured emergency response systems, chain of command medical logistics, and organized field care. He transitioned from the military to Seattle, Washington, where he joined the faculty at the University of Washington as a cardiologist and professor of medicine.

> Dr. Leonard Cobb knew that *everyone* could be a lifesaver.

In the 1960s, Dr. Cobb observed that most cardiac arrests occurred outside of hospitals, with no medically trained personnel close by, and survival rates were extremely low. He recognized that cardiac arrest survival was a *systems* problem, and he ap-

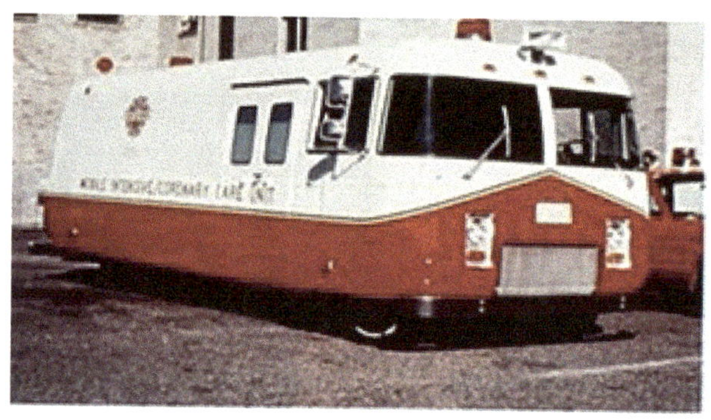

proached cardiac arrest death as a public health systems failure. He acknowledged that firefighters arrive on the scene to help patients long before they are seen by physicians. Therefore, he rationalized that educating the first responders was critical. They became the system of delivery.

Dr. Cobb's concepts were methodical, and they focused on measurable improvement. He insisted on data collection and producing quantifiable outcomes. He prioritized community CPR training, and he integrated firefighters, paramedics, physicians, and citizens into one coordinated survival network.

The Seattle Fire Department was open to physician oversight, and in 1969, Dr. Cobb partnered with them as their medical director, although the term had not yet been defined. They trained Medic One firefighters in Advanced Life Support, specifically for cardiac arrest, including high-quality CPR, manual defibrillation, cardiac rhythm interpretation, IV initiation, airway management, including intubation, and cardiac medicine administration.

Initially, the Medic One firefighters were a test group of 15 firefighters to determine if the radical idea of having advanced cardiac care performed by non-physicians under physician direction could work. The original Medic One unit was a motorhome converted into a mobile coronary unit. The early firefighter-paramedics nicknamed it "Moby Pig," a reference to its large size and speed.

Moby Pig operated out of Harborview Medical Center. It carried a defibrillator, cardiac monitor, oxygen, airway equipment, and medications, and it allowed the specially trained firefighters to deliver advanced cardiac care under physician direction. In the beginning, this unit arrived separate of other units. When it returned to the hospital, it bypassed the emergency department entirely.

In contrast to Dr. Cobb's foresight was the climate of that era. A 1966 National Academy of Sciences article titled *Accidental Death and Disability: The Neglected Disease of Modern Society* highlighted the inconsistencies with trauma response and the increase of trauma-related deaths, the *leading* cause of death, especially in younger populations. Although the report focused on trauma, the deficiencies it identified, delayed response, lack of training, and absence of coordinated prehospital care, applied equally to cardiac arrest, where survival depends on immediate intervention. The report exposed systemic gaps that also affected cardiac arrest survival, where delays in care often proved fatal.

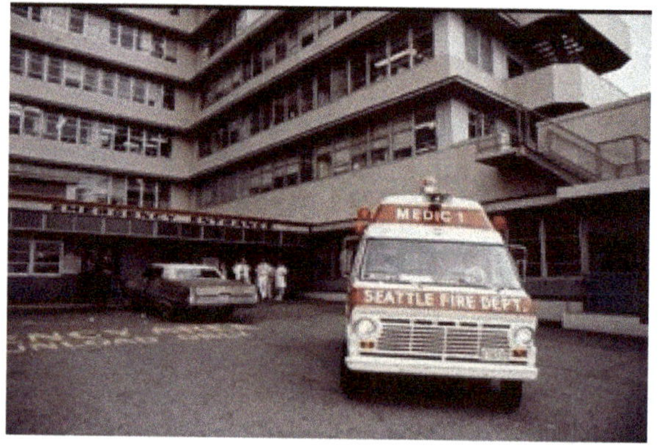

As data emerged from hospital research and early EMS systems, particularly in Seattle, it became clear that survival from ventricular fibrillation depended not on new treatments, but on delivering existing ones—CPR and defibrillation—before hospital arrival. The same delays that cost trauma patients their lives also proved fatal in cardiac arrest, where survival depends upon rapid, prehospital intervention.

Back then, the emergency response system was fragmented, and the level of care one received varied a lot by zip code. There were no national standards for response or training nor oversight. During an emergency, people called the operator (this was before 911), then they were patched directly through to the police or fire department.

Back then, most ambulances were operated by funeral homes because they had the equipment and the availability. However, the funeral homes did not have medical skills. The focus was on *transportation*—quickly getting a patient to medical professionals, not providing any care en route. Even firefighters only provided basic first aid.

The National Academy of Sciences article drew attention to these deficits and called these preventable occurrences a national public health crisis.

Although back then most cities had no formalized emergency medical services, a few cities *were* addressing the care deficits. In the early 1960s, in Miami, Florida, Dr. Eugene, "Gene" Nagel had the idea that firefighters could provide at-the-scene lifesaving care. He walked into the Miami Fire Department and began implementing the idea. By 1963, he was the Medical Director for the Miami Fire Department Rescue Division. He began teaching firefighters CPR, and he expanded firefighter training to include advanced airway management.

Concurrently during the 1960s, Dr. Nagel also developed a system linking field responders to hospital-based physicians via radio telemetry. Radio telemetry allowed paramedics to transmit cardiac rhythms and communicate directly with physicians in real time. This extended the reach of the hospital into the field. It enabled advanced medical care to begin before the patient ever arrived at the hospital.

This evolved into Rescue 1, a modified ambulance-type rescue vehicle operated by the Miami Fire Department, staffed by firefighters trained to provide care at the scene. Equipped with oxygen, airway tools, and radio communication, Rescue 1 represented a shift from transport-only ambulances toward vehicles capable of delivering prehospital treatment. Rescue 1 functioned as a mobile intensive care unit. It brought cardiac care directly to patients because it was also equipped with cardiac monitoring, defibrillation capability, advanced airway tools, IV medication, and radio-telemetry communication with physicians. This was one of the first times, if not *the* first time, that coronary care unit capability was bought into the field.

Among other major developments, Rescue 1 transmitted electrocardiogram (ECG) recordings from the field to hospital physicians, using radio-telemetry communication, which allowed physicians to supervise care and provide medical direction remotely. This shift was critical because responders could begin collecting meaningful medical *data* at the scene—rather than relying solely on visible symptoms. By placing electrodes on the patient's chest, paramedics could see the heart's electrical activity as a waveform on a monitor, allowing them and physicians via telemetry to identify lethal rhythms like ventricular fibrillation and act immediately.

People often say "radio telemetry" like it's one thing, but it's actually: telemetry (data) plus radio (voice) working together over radio frequencies. Rather than placing a physician in every ambulance, this model created a scalable system in which trained responders could deliver advanced care under physician supervision via radio.

Dr. Nagel linked the system by forging a practical, operational connection between three components that had previously functioned independently: firefighters, ambulances, and physicians. Before Nagel's work, the system was fragmented, firefighters responded to emergencies but provided minimal care, ambulances primarily served as transport vehicles, and physicians remained confined to the hospital. The three groups had little to no communication and no coordinated approach to patient care before arrival at the hospital. Nagel changed this by connecting the field to the hospital. As Medical Director, Dr. Nagel helped establish Miami's early fire-rescue system.

At the same time, Dr. Nagel established a receiving system within the hospital. Physicians were designated to monitor incoming calls and interpret transmitted data, and equipment was put in place to receive ECG signals via radio telemetry while maintaining two-way voice communication. This required the hospital to be actively engaged in prehospital care, prepared not just to receive patients, but to listen, interpret, and respond in real time.

The true link came together through the communication protocol Nagel developed. Firefighters would assess the patient, attach ECG leads when available, and begin immediate care such as CPR, airway management, and oxygen administration. Then they would contact the hospital via radio, transmitting or describing the patient's cardiac rhythm and overall condition. The physician would receive both data and verbal updates, evaluate the situation, ask clarifying questions, and issue explicit treatment orders.

This fundamentally changed the role of the responder. Firefighters were no longer acting independently; they were operating under direct physician supervision, albeit remotely. This required a new level of trust, clearly defined roles, and a repeatable process that could be relied upon in high-stress situations.

It also introduced something that had not previously existed in emergency response: a continuous feedback loop. Physicians could adjust treatment decisions in real time, and responders could immediately report changes in the patient's condition, creating an ongoing exchange rather than a single handoff. Dr. Nagel transformed emergency care from a disconnected sequence of actions into a coordinated system, where the field and the hospital functioned as extensions of one another and lifesaving care could begin at the scene.

Rescue 1's operational model provided further evidence that field defibrillation and physician-directed remote supervision worked. Together, the University of Miami, the Miami Fire Department, and Jackson Memorial Hospital proved that firefighters could be trained in advanced medical care and that telemetry could be used prehospital arrival. Rescue 1 laid the groundwork for modern Emergency Medical System (EMS) medical control systems.

Eugene "Gene" Nagel was born in 1924 in Clinton, Missouri, during the Great Depression. He grew up to serve in the US Army Signal Corps in the European Theater during World War II. His military communication system exposure would later influence his development of radio-based medical control in prehospital emergency care.

Following the war in 1949, Nagel earned an electrical engineering degree from Cornell University and set off into an electrical engineering career. He soon realized that was not his calling and attended the Washington University School of Medicine in St. Louis, where he earned his MD in 1959. He completed his residency at Columbia Presbyterian Medical Center in New York, with a specialty in anesthesiology, from 1959 to 1962. That's where Dr. Nagel became an early expert in the newly emerging CPR. Later in 1962, he joined the University of Miami School of Medicine as a faculty anesthesiologist.

> Dr. Eugene "Gene" Nagel recognized that firefighters *could* bring rapid care to a medical emergency—and save many lives.

A moment of enlightenment fell upon Dr. Nagel when a neighbor in his apartment building suffered cardiac arrest. The Miami firefighters unsuccessfully attempted resuscitation, then allegedly they told Dr. Nagel, "This always happens."

Dr. Nagel realized that would typically be the case, given the basic tools and skills the firefighters were equipped with. He also recognized that firefighters *could* bring rapid care to a medical emergency—and save many lives.

Although Rescue 1 was groundbreaking, globally speaking Dr. Frank Pantridge, a cardiologist from Belfast, Northern Ireland, is credited for creating the first mobile coronary unit in 1965, along with his colleague Dr. John Geddes, a cardiologist and physiologist.

I wanted to mention that sometimes it's hard to ascertain who actually did what first. Sometimes it comes down to who *published* it first. It's also hard to say whose work influenced what other work.

Dr. Pantridge's work was documented as inspiring at least two mobile coronary units in the United States. I also think the contributions Dr. Pantridge and Dr. Geddes made to the portable defibrillator were what really ignited an important shift in emergency care, making it possible to treat cardiac arrest in the field rather than relying solely on hospital-based interventions.

Prior to Dr. Pantridge and Dr. Geddes, defibrillators weighed more than 200 pounds and needed wall power. In Vietnam, the US military used early portable, battery-powered direct current (DC) defibrillators built around capacitor technology. Capacitor technology allows a defibrillator to store electrical energy and release it rapidly in a controlled burst, making it possible to deliver an effective shock to the heart. These defibrillators allowed defibrillation to be performed in the field and transport environments without reliance on fixed power sources. Simply put, without wall power.

Dr. Pantridge and Dr. Geddes developed a defibrillator weighing 150 pounds and able to fit inside an ambulance and run off of automobile batteries. That first defibrillator is said to have actually used *two* car batteries. The doctors published their work in the influential, international medical journal *The Lancet* in 1967 in an article titled, "A Mobile Intensive-Care Unit in the Management of Myocardial Infarction."

That article received global physician readership, rapid dissemination of information, and credibility—even for a controversial concept. That paper jump-started prehospital cardiac care *worldwide*, and within a few years, other cities created their own mobile coronary care units.

Another location that was greatly inspired by cardiac arrests and traumatic emergencies was Los Angeles, California. In the 1960s, LA had built the modern freeway system—generating high rates of freeway car crashes and traffic trauma. The city also had a lot of industrial accidents, burns, and construction injuries—plus, violence and shootings.

Harbor General Hospital, the county hospital and major trauma receiving center for Los Angeles County, was a teaching hospital affiliated with the University of California, Los Angeles School of Medicine. It later became known as Harbor-UCLA Medical Center. That hospital cared for patients with trauma injuries who were transported there by Los Angeles emergency responders. Sadly, patients arriving at the hospital in critical condition after receiving little to no treatment during transportation had a decreased rate of survival.

Before the formalization of emergency medical services' roles, terminology for clinicians varied widely, "ambulance attendant" was the most commonly used term in legal and regulatory language. The lack of a standardized or formally recognized prehospital provider role meant that people often operated under loosely defined expectations, performing a range of duties without a unified scope of practice, or title. Terminology varied widely, with terms such as ambulance driver, driver-attendant, ambulance aide, and rescue personnel used alongside "ambulance attendant," highlighting the lack of a unified or formally defined prehospital role. The workers had different scopes of practice, designed most likely by whoever paid them. Firefighters often were trained in basic first aid, but the others' training varied *a lot.*

To make matters worse, back then California law *prohibited* ambulance attendants and firefighters from providing anything beyond basic first aid and transport. However, the laws were not designed to be prohibitive. They were actually there to protect people from untrained individuals doing whatever they wanted. A Medical Practice Act is a state law that defines who is legally allowed to practice medicine and what that includes. State Medical Practice Acts restricted the practice of medicine to licensed physicians, leaving ambulance attendants and the like without legal authority to perform advanced care. Although Medical Practice Acts existed in every state, their interpretation and enforcement were not uniform, creating variability in what prehospital providers or ambulance attendants were able to do in practice. In some cases, the boundaries of allowable care were tested, highlighting the need for clearer legal frameworks.

People were dying in transport, *before* they even had a chance to receive treatment, *before* they arrived at the hospital. Fortunately, the National Academy of Sciences, National Research Council published *Accidental Death and Disability: The Neglected Disease of Modern Society* in 1966. The report is often referred to as a "white paper," a term used for authoritative government documents intended to guide policy and drive institutional change. It exposed critical failures in emergency care and helped ignite the development of modern emergency medical services systems.

With the white paper freshly published, institutions such as Harbor General Hospital explored ways to address these problems. Firefighters *already* communicated with hospital physicians and medical staff during patient handoff. Their communication soon evolved into collaboration. Then the Harbor-UCLA Medical Center and the Los Angeles County Fire Department petitioned lawmakers for legislation that would allow specially trained personnel to perform medical procedures under physician supervision. First responders would no longer be hamstringed by those old laws preventing them from providing more than basic first aid and transport.

The Los Angeles County Fire Department's network of fire stations responded rapidly to emergencies and was accustomed to operating within coordinated emergency response structures. They began deploying paramedics within the county system. Then county leaders approached state legislators. The ensuing bill defined what procedures paramedics *could* perform, their training requirements, physician oversight mechanisms, and how the hospital would supervise paramedics.

Those specifications became the basis for the Wedworth-Townsend Paramedic Act of 1970. Now paramedics communicated with physicians through radio systems connecting field units to Harbor General Hospital. Physicians authorized treatments, gave medical direction, and even provided real-time guidance during patient care. The paramedics were trained in airway management, defibrillation, electrocardiographic monitoring, intravenous therapy, medication administration, and trauma stabilization.

The Los Angeles paramedic program was born during a period when emergency medicine was emerging as a medical discipline. Hospitals were beginning to establish emergency departments and trauma care systems. Three physicians are credited with spearheading the rollout of this training program: Dr. Walter S. Graf, who significantly contributed to the development of paramedic education and medical oversight for prehospital care; Dr. J. Michael Criley, a cardiologist who focused on cardiovascular disease and acute cardiac emergencies; and Dr. Ronald D. Stewart, a specialist in emergency medicine and trauma care who participated in paramedic training development and emergency medical system development.

Those three doctors created protocols for medical guidance, treatment authorization, and oversight of prehospital care by doctors via paramedics in the field. These revolutionary concepts allowed for prehospital care to be effectively given under physician direction. They influenced EMS systems development throughout the United States, molding the paramedic profession during the late 1960s and early 1970s.

From a legal standpoint, Los Angeles county became one of the first places to attempt to solve the problem of people not receiving immediate medical care while in transport, allowing trained individuals to provide this care while en route before they reached the hospital. Having legislation geared toward emergency care was a major advancement. It showed other municipalities how it could be achieved.

Although Dr. Nagel formed the first US mobile intensive care unit, and California enacted the first legislature specifying what would become paramedic care, Dr. Cobb formally established the first comprehensive cardiac arrest registry and intervention program: The Seattle Heart Watch program.

This program was created to systematically track every out-of-hospital cardiac arrest in the Seattle area, study survival outcomes, improve EMS response times, promote widespread citizen CPR training, and integrate early defibrillation into prehospital care. It functioned as both a cardiac arrest occurrence registry and a systems-improvement initiative.

The city of Seattle was the ideal environment for this program due to its progressive fire department leadership and its strong partnership with the University of Washington. To create the Seattle Heart Watch Program, Dr. Cobb went to the Seattle Fire Department for collaboration, most likely with Chief Gordon Vickery. He and his colleagues were supportive of Dr. Cobb's philosophies. There was already an interest in expanding emergency medical services, and there was political support for paramedic development.

Dr. Cobb, the Seattle Fire Department, and regional medical leaders examined EMS response times, survival outcomes, and the impact of early CPR. Seattle Heart Watch tracked the outcomes of the interventions of *the Medic One initiative.* Remember them? The paramedics were trained to provide critical, lifesaving interventions, especially for cardiac emergencies, before the patient reached the hospital. This data could be measured and quantified. In essence, the fire department would respond to an emergency, the paramedics would treat the emergency, *Heart Watch* would measure, the data would allow for system improvements, and the cycle could be repeated again and again. The proof was in the pudding: Medic One delivered the care, and Seattle Heart Watch proved the care worked. This was a game-changer.

Dr. Cobb and his colleagues documented survival rates for ventricular fibrillation, (VF) a chaotic heart rhythm that can be reversed with defibrillation, at less than 5 percent. In Seattle, however, survival improved to 20 to 40 percent in cases where the arrest was witnessed, a shockable rhythm was present, and rapid response times allowed for early intervention.

Harborview Medical Center was the medical hub of Seattle Heart Watch and trained and oversaw the Medic One paramedics. The hospital provided medical leadership, and Dr. Cobb and his colleagues implemented protocols and treatment guidelines. The earliest Seattle paramedics trained at Harborview under physician supervision and contacted physicians by radio for treatment orders. The data gathered by Seattle Heart Watch was analyzed and published across multiple peer-reviewed medical journals, including early reports in the *American Journal of Cardiology* in the 1970s, with ongoing analyses appearing in *Circulation* and the *Journal of the American College of Cardiology.*

This data clarified several important things. First, VF was the main cause of sudden cardiac arrest death. Second, rapid defibrillation was crucial to increasing cardiac arrest survival. Third, a patient's chances of surviving cardiac arrest dropped dramatically with each passing minute without treatment. Fourth, bystander CPR before paramedics arrive improved survival. These findings later influenced the global resuscitation strategy.

Because of Dr. Cobb's work, Seattle developed a system where cardiac arrests were carefully tracked, paramedics were medically trained and supervised, citizens were trained in CPR, and outcomes were scientifically measured.

Between 1962 and 1970, a cluster of early mobile cardiac care experiments were performed. These systems all aimed to treat cardiac arrest and heart attack before the patient reached the hospital, even if they were not specifically cardiac focused. Some of these ambulance style services are less mentioned, but they were crucial in the roles that they played and the knowledge that they gleaned from their work.

In 1967, the Freedom House Ambulance service was created in conjunction with the University of Pittsburgh by Dr. Peter Safar, mentioned earlier as the Father of CPR, and Dr. Nancy Caroline, an American physician educated at Barnard College and the University of Pittsburgh. In 1968, the Freedom House Ambulance service began full ambulance operations—the first US ambulance service that was staffed by paramedics whose extensive training exceeded basic first aid and included advanced airway management, CPR, IV therapy, cardiac care, plus emergency medical technician training, including patient assessment, oxygen therapy, emergency child birthing, splinting, trauma care, anatomy, and pharmacology. The ambulance also carried actual medical equipment.

> In 1968, the Freedom House Ambulance service began full ambulance operations—the first US ambulance service that was staffed by paramedics whose extensive training exceeded basic first aid.

American race relations of the time most likely hindered the popularity of this ambulance team because most of the crew members were African-American males from the Hill District, a historically significant Black neighborhood in Pittsburgh known for its rich cultural legacy and the lasting impact of urban renewal. Still, the Freedom House Ambulance service's innovative emergency care emerged within that underserved community, where gaps in emergency care were both visible and urgent. The program focused on training community members as paramedics and providing emergency medical care in the field. Some of those trained had faced previous employment obstacles and had limited opportunities.

The Freedom House Ambulance service is often regarded as one of the first modern paramedic services in the United States. It demonstrated that non-physicians could deliver advanced emergency care in the field, and it contributed to modern paramedic programs. Studies conducted at the time found that the Freedom House Ambulance teams provided higher quality care than many other existing ambulance services, above expected prehospital treatment for cardiac and trauma patients, and performed complex emergency care outside hospitals.

Despite its success, the Freedom House Ambulance service faced political resistance, and in the 1970s, it was replaced by a city-run EMS system. Most of the original Freedom House Ambulance personnel were not employed by the new municipal service. That decision, which was likely motivated by prejudice, later earned some criticism. Nevertheless, the Freedom House Ambulance service is widely recognized as a major milestone in EMS development.

In the early 1970s, Dr. Nancy Caroline became the medical director for the Freedom House Ambulance Service. She was responsible for designing paramedic training curriculum, supervising field protocols, and ensuring clinical standards for emergency care. Later, she wrote one of the most influential paramedic textbooks, *Emergency Care in the Streets,* which became a standard reference for paramedic education. She later went abroad to help develop international EMS systems, including programs in Israel.

Around that same time, in 1968, another notable mobile coronary care unit operated in New York City under the medical leadership of Dr. William Grace at St. Vincent's Hospital. This mobile unit featured physician-staffed ambulances and cardiac monitoring and defibrillation capability. The goal was to treat lethal arrhythmia before hospital arrival. The project was partially funded through federal Regional Medical Program grants. This was modeled directly after the work of cardiologists Dr. Frank Pantridge and Dr. John Geddes who led the Belfast work and brought us the first portable defibrillator.

Come 1969, under the medical direction of Dr. James Warren and Dr. Richard Lewis, associated with the Ohio State University and in collaboration with the Columbus Fire Department, the Columbus Heartmobile was created. It featured a paramedic-based cardiac ambulance, ECG monitoring, and prehospital treatment for myocardial infarction. Initially it was staffed by specially trained firefighters, who would later become paramedics, and an attending physician.

Soon, researchers realized that trained emergency ambulance crews could deliver the care independent of a physician, and by 1971 physicians stopped riding in the ambulances. It became an ambulance personnel-run system, which influenced EMS nationwide.

Dr. Pantridge's findings influenced one of the earliest examples of rural EMS organization and execution. In Haywood County, North Carolina, a team of mobile intensive care technicians were supervised by Dr. Ralph Feichter, an internal medicine physician in Waynesville, North Carolina, who served as the Medical Director for the Haywood County Volunteer Rescue Squad Program. That volunteer rescue squad was comprised of specially trained emergency personnel and mobile intensive care vehicles. Dr. Feichter trained approximately 40 volunteers in cardiac physiology, defibrillation, CPR, and advanced emergency care. The group acquired funding for two mobile intensive care vehicles.

Together, the efforts of Freedom House Ambulance service, Rescue 1, the New York mobile coronary unit, Columbus Heartmobile, Haywood County's mobile intensive care technicians, the LA Fire Department, and Dr. Cobb's movement drove the organization of EMS systems across the United States. These programs proved that paramedics were well equipped to provide advanced emergency care. By that time, more communities had access to advanced care outside of the hospital. This increased the likelihood of survival after sudden cardiac arrest.

However, despite advances in resuscitation, sudden cardiac arrest remains a major public health problem to this day, with high incidence, low survival, and significant dependence on timely bystander intervention. As of 2020, according to the American Heart Association (AHA), approximately 356,000 out-of-hospital cardiac arrests occur each year in the United States. Survival decreases by approximately 7 to 10 percent for *every minute* without intervention. Survival to discharge is around 10 percent.

Although only about 40 percent of patients receive bystander CPR, those who do are *two to three times* more likely to survive. With early defibrillation in public settings, survival can approach 40 to 50 percent.

> Although only about 40 percent of patients receive bystander CPR, those who do are two to three times more likely to survive. With early defibrillation in public settings, survival can approach 40 to 50 percent.

Here are two important takeaways: Military medics and anesthesiologists played big parts in shaping the US Emergency Medical System. Medics had experience stabilizing patients before evacuation, which later influenced emergency care. Anesthesiologists are the physicians most experienced with airway management, ventilation, oxygen delivery, and resuscitation physiology.

We talked about Medic One, and you might be wondering about Medic Two, who are lay persons trained to respond to emergencies. It took all of these steps, and much more, to get to the point where the masses could be trained. First, we needed the science, then we needed the proof that it actually worked, and then we needed people to understand how it worked and to be able to apply that knowledge in the field.

Data from Seattle Heart Watch made it crystal clear that early intervention during cardiac arrest was critical in increasing survival rates. The chance of survival declines every minute without CPR, so bystander CPR was the solution.

In 1972 in Seattle, Dr. Cobb and Seattle Fire Chief Gordon Vickery launched the world's first mass citizen CPR training program. Dr. Cobb was motivated by the data that showed that early intervention saved lives. By empowering regular citizens to act quickly, he helped reshape emergency care. This venture aggressively trained teachers, police officers, airport personnel, office workers, non-paramedic firefighters, and even ordinary citizens in CPR. In Medic Two's first two years, more than 100,000 people were trained, and it became the model for public CPR instruction.

Interestingly, even in the 1970s, there was no standard word for "paramedic" yet. (I know, I used the term throughout this book, but it was for simplicity's sake.) No one is exactly sure who was the first to use the word. Some say Dr. Eugene "Gene" Nagel of Miami, but others say he used the terminology "mobile intensive care unit attendant" or "paramedical staff." The point is that the terms were not standardized during this time, but because Dr. Nagel had his mobile ambulance service trials in the early 1960s, he likely was a contributing factor.

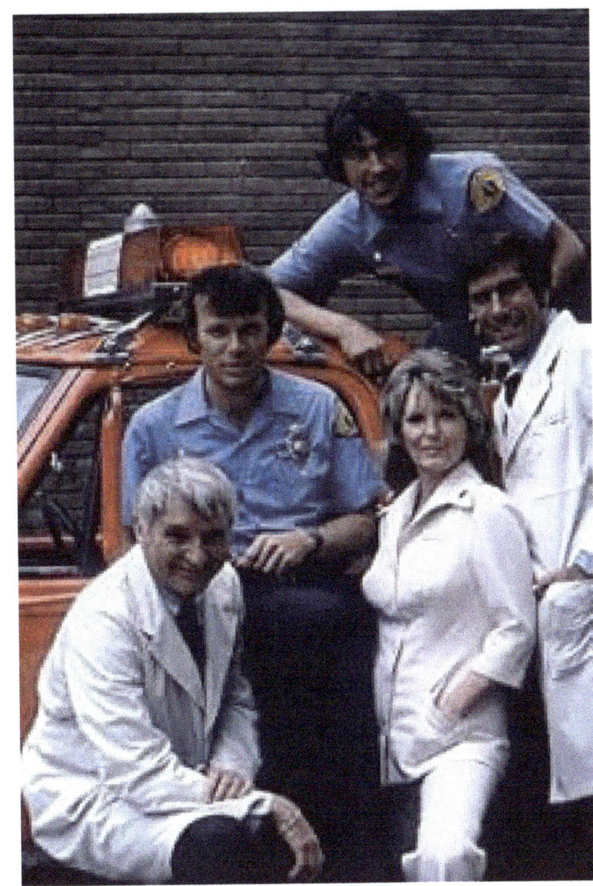

Dr. Cobb might have used terms like "emergency medical technician" or "firefighter-medic," or he might have described people with advanced skills. Early documentation of the profession says "firefighters trained in advanced life support" or "mobile intensive care personnel."

Ironically, the two things that solidified the use of the term "paramedic" were the Los Angeles County legislature utilizing it and the 1972 show *Emergency!* That show was inspired by the Los Angeles paramedics program, and it depicted firefighters trained as paramedics delivering advanced emergency care in the field. Despite being scripted and dramatized, the program educated the public on the new paramedic profession, and it increased support for emergency medical systems throughout the United States.

Emergency! was created by Robert A. Cinader and Jack Webb. Cinader came up with the show concept when he visited the fire department and was introduced to the new paramedics program and physicians at Harbor General Hospital. Later, Cinader used that knowledge to convince television producers of the legitimacy and necessity of the show's message. Allegedly, the producers did not believe that this was a real profession. However, once they were shown paramedic training, fire department rescue squads, advanced emergency procedure demos, defibrillation, cardiac monitoring, IV therapy, and airway management, the NBC pilot was approved. The rest is a wrap!

Emergency! aired from 1972 through 1977, highlighting the firefighter-paramedics working for the Los Angeles County Fire Department. The series portrayed a medical rescue squad assigned to a fire station, which responded to accidents, fires, and other medical emergencies. Episodes generally illustrated a call being received by dispatch operators, then the rescue squad responding with treatment at the scene and transporting to a hospital emergency department.

The main characters were Johnny Gage and Roy DeSoto, primary paramedics responding to events in the field and at the hospital. Dr. Kelly Brackett oversaw emergency care with support from nurse Dixie McCall and other hospital support staff. The production worked extremely closely with the Los Angeles Fire Department and Harbor General Hospital to create very accurate reenactments in their series. Both Cinader and Webb took attention to detail and accuracy very seriously.

Interestingly, real firefighters and paramedics appeared on the show. Mike Stoker and Marco Lopez were actual Los Angeles County firefighters, and Dick Hammer was a Battalion Chief with the Los Angeles County Fire Department.

The show dramatically increased public awareness of emergency medical systems and the paramedics profession. This greatly disseminated the idea that lifesaving treatment could begin before a patient even reached a hospital. Many other communities began envisioning rescue units incorporating paramedics for their residents.

Many firefighters who entered EMS in the 1970s and the 1980s cite *Emergency!* as their inspiration for entering the profession. For many people, the show was their introduction to emergency paramedicine and CPR.

Show Cinader began personally promoting EMS after he saw how impactful the show had become. He advocated for public CPR training and emergency preparedness. He worked to increase awareness of paramedic services, and he supported national EMS conferences and events advocating for CPR education, paramedic system development, and recognition of lifesaving responders. Even after the show left syndication, Cinader used television to educate the public about lifesaving skills.

It was becoming more accepted that rapid EMS saves lives. That knowledge combined with the Seattle Heart Watch data that demonstrated that early CPR saves lives, the fact that early defibrillation saves lives, and the concept that systems measurement improves survival. The American Heart Association (AHA) created CPR programs that reflected paramedic system development, AED public access initiatives, cardiac arrest registries, and the modern Chain of Survival framework. This evolved into the four original links in the Chain of Survival:

early access, early CPR, early defibrillation, and early advanced care, which contributed to the foundation of the Resuscitation Academy.

In the 1970s, CPR was becoming standard in cardiac circles and emergency medical care. Now we had CPR and organizations teaching CPR, but *which* CPR were they teaching?

Back then, researchers and clinicians frequently disagreed on the *correct* methods for resuscitation. Recommendations varied for compression depth, compression rate, breathing techniques, and sequencing of intervention steps.

But to increase bystander CPR participation, potential bystanders needed to be trained on CPR. And to train bystanders on CPR, experts needed to simplify and standardize it.

Other obstacles to training the public on CPR back then included people's uncertainty about CPR's effectiveness. Adoption by the public was slow, so the National Academy of Sciences (NAS) convened a major conference on resuscitation in 1966.

The NAS is an independent scientific advisory council to the US government. Expert panelists assemble to investigate major national problems, then they publish reports that influence policy decisions in engineering, medicine, and science.

You might recall that the NAS published the *Accidental Death and Disability: The Neglected Disease of Modern Society*. That was one of the NAS's most ground-breaking contributions to emergency medicine. The report showed that emergency medical services in the United States were severely fragmented. Ambulance attendants had minimal training, and emergency communication systems were not unified, but the biggest concern was that survival from trauma and cardiac arrest was poor. The report recommended improved training of personnel, expanded resuscitation techniques, improved ambulance systems, national standards for emergency care, and development of a national emergency medical system. That report was a major catalyst for change regarding emergency medical care, which was a good thing because the current model was dangerously inadequate.

With no national authority officiating on how CPR should be taught, several groups began doing their own thing. Hospitals taught physicians, fire departments trained responders, the Red Cross taught the public first aid, and medical researchers published the evolving techniques.

The NAS ignited the situation with a conference on resuscitation in 1966, and by the time the conference adjourned, they had created the first national standard recommendations for CPR and training. The NAS asked the AHA to lead the standardization of CPR so that everyone would be able to be taught the same things.

By this time, the AHA was already a major national organization focused on cardiovascular disease research and physician education. Remember it was an organization initially comprised of cardiologists. By the time of this conference, the AHA had a national network of physicians and cardiologists, and it had established scientific conferences, publication systems, and an infrastructure to disseminate education to physicians. Because cardiac arrest is fundamentally a cardiovascular event, cardiologists and cardiac researchers had been working with the AHA for decades, and CPR right along with it. This gave the organization the influence and position to coordinate the emerging science of CPR, training, and standardization.

Many hospitals and physicians of the time trusted the clinical guidance provided by the AHA because of its cardiovascular data and the fact that sites with the first emergency mobile units that incorporated CPR were often affiliated with the AHA. Thus, the industry leaders were previously affiliated with the AHA, who had funded and supported a lot of research. The AHA was zealous in the advancement of cardiac care, even before CPR was formalized. The national cardiology research community was well represented in the AHA, so it seemed like a natural fit.

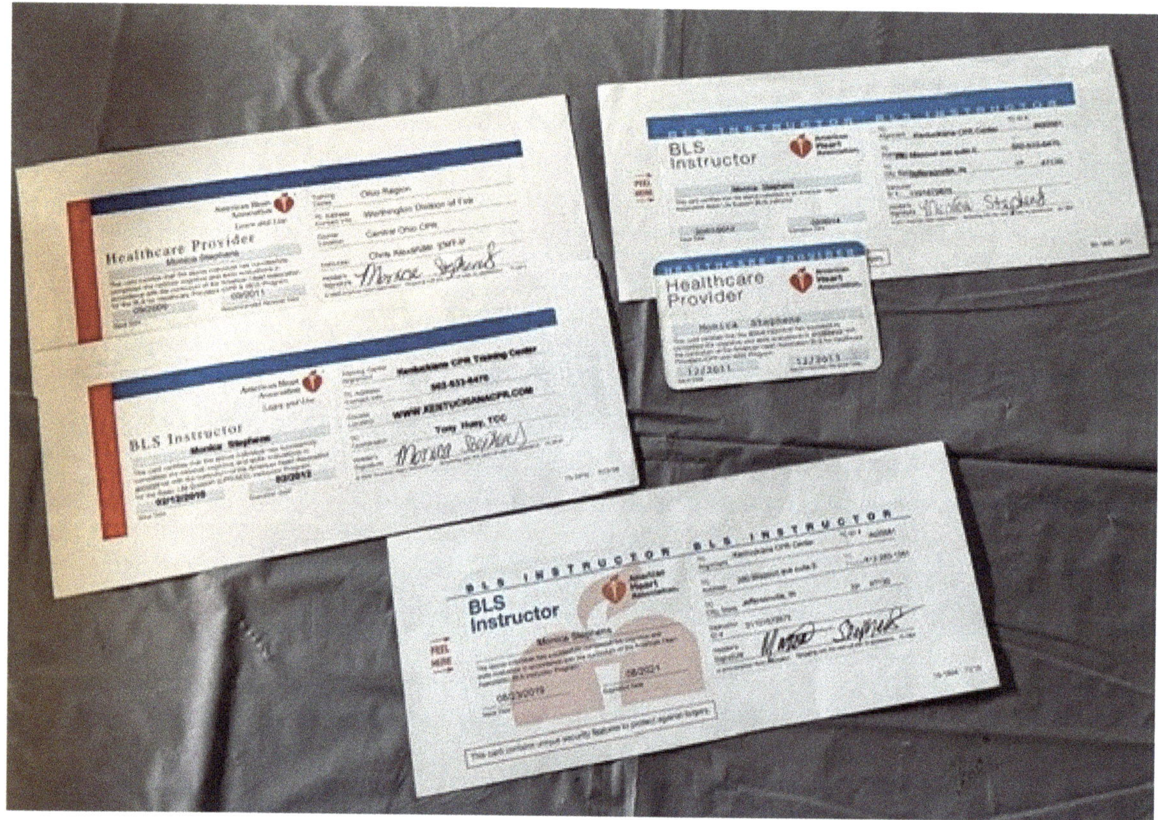

The AHA then began convening conferences on cardiopulmonary resuscitation and emergency cardiac care, and it published standardized recommendations. The science eventually developed into the Emergency Cardiac Care system, which includes Basic Life Support (BLS), defibrillation protocols, Advanced Cardiac Life Support (ACLS), Pediatric Advanced Life Support (PALS), and national instructor training courses.

The AHA produces national clinical guidelines for cardiac care, maintains physician networks and cardiology leadership, and influences hospital training standards and national training programs.

You might have already suspected this: The selection of the AHA to standardize CPR did not sit well with all other organizations. For example, the American Red Cross, which was founded in 1881 by Clara Barton after her experiences providing care during the Civil War, had taught first aid and lifesaving courses for decades before modern CPR had materialized and organized. The Red Cross already had national instructor networks, training materials, public trust, and government partnerships. In the 1960s, the Red Cross incorporated CPR into its community training program.

Scan to hear from the American Red Cross.

Alas, there was a bit of friction between the AHA and the Red Cross about whose curriculum should be used, whose certification should be acknowledged, and which organization would dominate CPR education. For years, the two organizations ran parallel CPR training systems, often with subtle differences. The Red Cross retained its own training system despite the AHA standardizing CPR, CPR instructor courses, and training centers. As a result, hospitals often followed AHA standards, community classes were often Red Cross, and fire departments chose one or the other. This created two national CPR ecosystems.

The paramedic push muddied the water even more. Back when paramedics had to be under physician direction, many of those physicians were aligned with the AHA and its training system. This further strengthened the AHA's influence, and it would eventually formalize a larger system, the Emergency Cardiovascular Care (ECC) system. Once the ECC became widely adopted in hospitals and EMS systems, the AHA gained scientific authority over resuscitation standards. Increasingly, other groups aligned with the AHA's guidelines.

Over time, the conflict neutralized. Maybe everyone realized that the point is to work together to get more people trained in CPR and lifesaving skills. It could definitely have been because CPR techniques became evidence-based. Once science was applied, the organizations began sharing and combining guidelines. There was instructor cross-training, and many instructors were certified to teach under different entities.

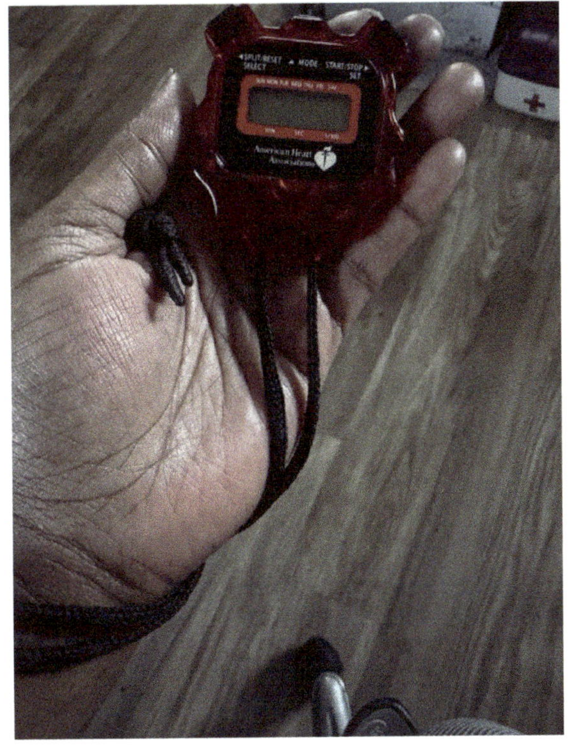

A practical division developed, which I experienced personally as an instructor. I initially instructed for the Red Cross and became a Pet First Aid instructor. I had thought I could become an American Red Cross instructor and gain reciprocity with the Red Cross. That is not what happened, but an opportunity presented for me to teach Pet First Aid. Today the AHA is the go-to for clinical research and science, clinical guidelines, healthcare provider training, and resuscitation standards. The Red Cross took the lead in community CPR training, first aid integration, and mass public interaction, in addition to all of the other things it does.

Despite the AHA and Red Cross's differences, the two organizations enabled CPR classes to be provided in workplaces, for firefighters and paramedics, and in schools. By the late 20th century, CPR had become a community skill, rather than just a medical procedure.

As more time passed, there was more global collaboration, and international research bodies helped to unify standards. The AHA was a major contributor to global review of CPR science through the International Liaison Committee on Resuscitation (ILCOR), which was established in 1992. This furthered the AHA's influence on resuscitation guidelines.

Somewhere in all of that, the AHA adopted the initial Chain of Survival concept:

1. Early recognition of cardiac arrest
2. Early CPR
3. Early defibrillation
4. Advanced care

This made CPR *part* of the emergency response system, instead of its own isolated technique.

It is also interesting to note that another piece of emergency response was emerging around this time: the Heimlich maneuver, which is also referred to as "abdominal thrusts." In the 1970s, choking was the sixth leading cause of accidental death in the United States, killing nearly 4,000 people each year. The numbers might have been even higher because often the deaths were classified as asphyxia or cardiac arrest. According to the *New York Times,* thoracic surgeon Dr. Henry Heimlich was struck by the fact that many choking deaths occurred because people mistook choking for a heart attack—a phenomenon known as a "café coronary." Back then, the standard response to choking was back blows—sharp strikes to the back that were widely taught but were often ineffective and worse could drive the obstruction deeper into the person's airway. The only alternative was a tracheostomy, an invasive surgical procedure requiring medical expertise. This left a dangerous gap between what bystanders could do and what physicians could provide.

> Through experiments on anesthetized dogs, Dr. Henry Heimlich developed a technique that he said "any informed layman" could use to help a person choking by giving a rapid upward thrust beneath the ribcage to harness the lungs' residual air and forcefully eject the obstruction—an effect he likened to a "small hurricane."

While Dr. Heimlich was working as a thoracic surgeon at Jewish Hospital in Cincinnati, he set out to close that gap by creating a method that "any informed layman" could use. Through experiments on anesthetized dogs, Dr. Heimlich developed a technique using a rapid upward thrust beneath the ribcage to harness the lungs' residual air and forcefully eject the obstruction—an effect he likened to a "small hurricane." He introduced the maneuver publicly in June 1974 in the journal *Emergency Medicine* in an article titled "Pop Goes the Café Coronary."

Within days of media coverage, Dr. Heimlich's technique was reportedly used by a bystander to save a choking victim, marking its first real-world application. Despite the Heimlich maneuver's rapid public uptake, Dr. Heimlich spent years in conflict with organizations such as the American Red Cross, which continued to recommend back blows as an initial response. Over time, the Heimlich maneuver gained broader institutional acceptance, and it became integrated into emergency response training as a central component of choking intervention in first aid practice.

As long as I have been an instructor, we have taught abdominal thrusts as part of Basic Life Support (BLS). That's why, I felt the need to include this tidbit. The Heimlich maneuver is not part of CPR, but if someone is choking, you might need to perform this maneuver to avoid having to do CPR. Ironically, the latest American Heart Association update added back blows to the abdominal thrusts.

Back to the AHA. By 1999, the AHA launched the Registry of Cardiopulmonary Resuscitation, one of the largest cardiac arrest research databases, to collect standardized hospital cardiac arrest data. This data allowed researchers to study CPR quality, survival trends, and other details that shaped future guideline updates.

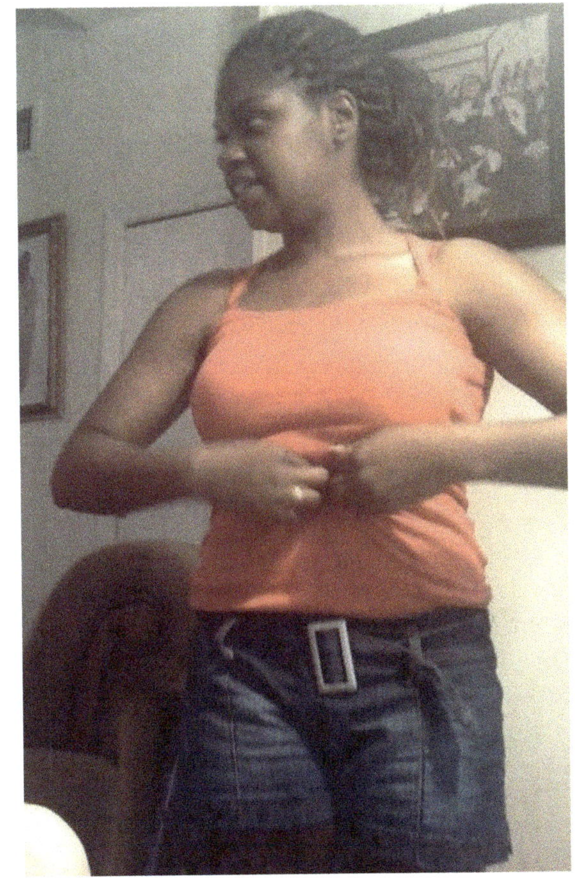

In 2010, the registry evolved into Get with the Guidelines—Resuscitation, a nationwide data system tracking in-hospital cardiac arrest outcomes. This is why we currently update our certifications every two years, and the AHA revises their recommendations every five years.

The AHA has also driven public CPR awareness campaigns, such as Hands-Only CPR. The push for compression-only CPR for untrained bystanders was part of the effort to increase intervention rates.

The AHA turned scattered research into clear national protocols and built an entire CPR education program, including training infrastructure, curriculum, certifications, and instructor networks to disseminate CPR science to the United States and the world. Today, the AHA serves as both a scientific authority on CPR research and the public education leader for CPR training. And CPR is a nationwide, public health intervention.

Chapter 5: The Beat Beyond Borders

Up to this point, we've mainly focused on the United States. However, the evolution of emergency care in the United States was part of a larger global movement. Before modern paramedicine, many countries relied on charitable, volunteer, or first aid organizations for emergency response. Among these were the St. John Ambulance Jamaica association (1899), the Cuban Red Cross (1909), the Mexican Red Cross (1910), and early organized ambulance corps in South Africa (1896).

Scan to learn more about the beat beyond borders.

These organizations provided some of the earliest coordinated emergency care systems, often combining first aid training with transportation to hospitals. Researchers, governments, and emergency response organizations were gradually recognizing the same reality: Survival from cardiac arrest depends on whether someone nearby knows what to do and how quickly help arrives. Despite lacking in advanced medical capability, pioneers like the St. John Ambulance created the foundation for coordinated emergency response that later evolved into modern Emergency Medical Services (EMS) systems.

By the mid-1900s, emergency response began shifting from transport-only services to medicalized prehospital systems. Governments and health organizations worldwide began developing formal EMS, introducing trained responders who were capable of providing lifesaving interventions *before* hospital arrival. Programs expanded across North America, Europe, Asia, and parts of Latin America and Africa. Countries introduced paramedic roles, national CPR training campaigns, and ambulance systems equipped to deliver oxygen, CPR, and eventually defibrillation in the field.

The development of EMS systems became increasingly critical because by the end of the 20th century, sudden cardiac arrest had emerged as one of the most significant public health challenges worldwide. Today, estimates suggest that millions of people worldwide experience sudden cardiac arrest each year, with approximately 350,000 out-of-hospital cardiac arrests occurring annually in the United States alone. In Canada, the number is estimated at around 60,000 cardiac arrests per year, while European countries report similar rates when adjusted for population.

> Despite advances in medicine, survival rates of out-of-hospital cardiac arrest remained low—often less than 10 percent overall in many regions during the late 20th century.

But research consistently yielded that survival increased dramatically when bystanders initiated CPR and when defibrillation occurred quickly.

During the late 20th century, defibrillation technology gradually moved beyond hospital operating rooms and coronary care units. Portable defibrillators began appearing in emergency departments and ambulances in the 1970s, allowing treatment for cardiac arrest to begin earlier in the chain of survival. By the 1980s and 1990s, defibrillator technology had improved, and several EMS systems around the world had integrated defibrillation into prehospital care. Examples include ambulance systems across North America, Europe, Asia, and Australia, Canada, United States, Singapore, and Japan.

These advancements allowed for defibrillation to begin in workplaces, public spaces, and even homes—rather than waiting for arrival at an emergency department. Resuscitation science had moved beyond individual researchers and hospital laboratories. CPR and defibrillation had become a global effort, coordinated across continents.

Despite these advances, approaches to cardiac arrest care varied significantly between countries. Differences in emergency infrastructure, training standards, and public awareness meant that survival outcomes differed widely across regions.

Researchers and medical organizations recognized that resuscitation science was advancing rapidly, but without global collaboration, the adoption of best practices would remain inconsistent. In 1989, the European Resuscitation Council (ERC) was established to develop CPR guidelines and training programs across Europe.

As research on resuscitation science accelerated globally during the late 1980s and early 1990s, leaders in the field increasingly recognized the need for international collaboration to evaluate evidence and coordinate guidelines. This led to one of the most important milestones in modern cardiac arrest response: the formation of the International Liaison Committee on Resuscitation (ILCOR) in 1992. This collaboration convened resuscitation councils from around the world to evaluate research and guide the future of CPR and defibrillation.

The ILCOR brought together several of the world's leading resuscitation organizations, including the American Heart Association in the United States, the European Resuscitation Council of Europe, the Heart and Stroke Foundation of Canada, the Australian and New Zealand Committee on Resuscitation, the Resuscitation Councils of Southern Africa, and the InterAmerican Heart Foundation, which represented Latin America and the Caribbean.

Each regional council contributed different strengths to the development of resuscitation science and education.

- The European Resuscitation Council helped advance large-scale cardiac arrest research and population registries across Europe, producing important data on survival outcomes and emergency response systems.
- The Heart and Stroke Foundation of Canada played a major role in expanding nationwide CPR education and integrating resuscitation training with emergency medical services research.
- The Australian and New Zealand Committee on Resuscitation contributed strong expertise in evidence-based guideline development and national policy for resuscitation and first aid education.

- The Resuscitation Council of Asia helped coordinate growing research and training initiatives across a large and diverse population, supporting the expansion of CPR education and public defibrillation programs.
- The Resuscitation Council of Southern Africa contributed perspectives on implementing resuscitation training and emergency care in regions with varied healthcare infrastructure, helping ensure that international recommendations could be applied in both resource-rich and resource-limited settings.
- The InterAmerican Heart Foundation worked to expand cardiovascular health education and CPR training initiatives throughout Latin America and the Caribbean.

ILCOR functions as an international nonprofit organization under Belgian law and brings together organizations responsible for developing resuscitation guidelines in different regions of the world. Member organizations generally represent multidisciplinary groups involved in resuscitation science, education, and clinical care. Through this international network, ILCOR provides a mechanism for reviewing scientific evidence and developing consensus on resuscitation practices. Its work has played an important role in aligning CPR and emergency cardiovascular care guidelines across countries and ensuring that advances in resuscitation science are evaluated collaboratively on a global scale.

ILCOR focuses mainly on evidence review. All member councils participate in evidence evaluation and consensus development, ensuring that resuscitation recommendations consider different healthcare systems and populations around the world. Researchers from participating councils evaluate new studies on topics such as CPR techniques, compression depth and rate, ventilation strategies, defibrillation timing, medications used during cardiac arrest, and post-resuscitation care.

Over time, ILCOR grew to include representatives from resuscitation councils across multiple regions of the world. Current member organizations include the American Heart Association (AHA), the Australian and New Zealand Committee on Resuscitation (ANZCOR), the Australian Resuscitation Council, the New Zealand Resuscitation Council, the European Resuscitation Council (ERC), the Heart and Stroke Foundation of Canada (HSFC), the InterAmerican Heart Foundation (IAHF), the Indian Resuscitation Council Federation (IRCF), the Resuscitation Council of Asia (RCA), and the Resuscitation Councils of Southern Africa (RCSA). Additionally, ILCOR collaborates with global humanitarian organizations, such as the International Federation of Red Cross and Red Crescent Societies (IFRC).

Within this global framework, ILCOR evaluates the scientific research related to resuscitation, while organizations like the AHA and ERC translate that evidence into formal training protocols and educational programs for healthcare providers and the public.

It is true that different parts of the world often follow guidelines issued by their own regional resuscitation councils; however, the underlying science *guiding* those recommendations is coordinated through ILCOR. In this way, organizations such as the AHA contribute to national training efforts and also to a broader global network working to improve survival from cardiac arrest through consistent, evidence-based resuscitation practices.

For example, the AHA has long played a central role in developing and disseminating CPR and emergency cardiovascular care training. In 1966, the AHA helped publish the first widely recognized national CPR training recommendations in the United States. During the 1970s, the organization built a standardized instructor training system and standardized CPR courses that could be taught consistently in hospitals, emergency services, and community programs. Because the AHA had developed a standardized instructor model and reproducible course materials, it was able to license international training centers that could teach these courses locally while maintaining the same curriculum and certification standards. Over time, this network allowed AHA training programs—such as Basic Life Support (BLS), Advanced Cardiovascular Life Support (ACLS), Pediatric Advanced Life Support (PALS), and Heartsaver courses—to expand to hospitals, universities, and community training centers in more than 100 countries, making them one of the most widely recognized resuscitation training systems in the world.

The international AHA programs are especially common in parts of Latin America, the Middle East, Asia, and Africa, where many healthcare institutions rely on AHA certification for professional credentialing. In Canada, AHA training has been used alongside programs developed by the Heart and Stroke Foundation, while some institutions in Europe and other regions incorporate AHA courses into their own regional training systems.

Another major contributing factor to the American Heart Association training curriculum spreading beyond the United States was the growing international standardization of hospital credentialing during the 1980s and 1990s. When advanced life support courses such as Advanced Cardiovascular Life Support (ACLS) were developed in the late 1970s and early 1980s, they quickly became recognized as a structured way to train physicians, nurses, and paramedics to manage cardiac arrest and other cardiovascular emergencies. Because the courses were based on detailed algorithms, standardized teaching materials, and formal instructor certification, hospitals could rely on them as a consistent benchmark for clinical competence. With international healthcare systems modernizing, many hospitals, especially in regions with strong U.S. affiliation, began requiring ACLS and Basic Life Support (BLS) certification for physicians, nurses, and emergency personnel.

This was particularly common in parts of the Middle East, Asia, and Latin America, where hospitals frequently trained staff using American residency programs, medical textbooks, or visiting faculty. In these settings, AHA courses became a convenient and widely recognized credential for demonstrating competency in resuscitation care.

In 2000, the first internationally coordinated CPR guidelines were published through ILCOR collaboration, helping align resuscitation science across countries while allowing each region to produce its own training programs. Different organizations face different challenges, such as limited resources, disease burden, EMS infrastructure, and different health prioritizations. Having the open channels of communication allowed for collaboration and ultimately more people trained in CPR.

While organizations such as the AHA led training and guideline development, large population research from Europe and collaborative clinical studies from North America provided data that shaped international resuscitation science. Combined, these developments reflect a gradual shift from isolated research efforts toward a coordinated global approach to resuscitation science.

Chapter 6: Carrying the Rhythm Forward

The science of resuscitation might have been debated in meeting rooms and refined through international guidelines, but its survival depended on something far simpler: the willingness of people to learn how to act.

Scan to learn more about Bob Kaplan and Memoirs of the CPR Industry.

By the time worldwide resuscitation organizations began outlining their guidelines, CPR was no longer confined to hospitals and medical professionals. Even though modern CPR was first standardized in the United States in the 1960s, prior contributions to resuscitation science—including mouth-to-mouth ventilation, bioelectric research, and defibrillation—emerged from Europe and other regions long before CPR became a thing.

Once CPR was formalized and taught at scale in the United States, other countries did not passively adopt it. Instead they adapted, refined, and expanded it within their own healthcare systems. The 1970s marked the beginning of widespread international CPR adoption. However, this expansion did not occur through a single global authority. Instead, CPR training developed independently across different countries, each adapting the technique to its own healthcare systems, resources, and culture. Many countries established their own resuscitation councils and developed training programs that reflected their local emergency response infrastructure.

From the 1970s through the 1990s, CPR education grew expeditiously around the world through public health campaigns and national training initiatives. Community classes, workplace programs, school-based instruction, and public service announcements helped shift CPR from a clinical skill to a shared social responsibility.

The pioneers of resuscitation discovered how to restart the human heart, but *instructors* would carry that knowledge into the classrooms, workplaces, and communities around the globe.

The pioneers of resuscitation discovered how to restart the human heart, but *instructors* would carry that knowledge into the classrooms, workplaces, and communities around the globe.

The United States is generally recognized for standardizing and scaling CPR training, particularly through organizations like the American Heart Association (AHA). However, other regions, especially in Europe and Scandinavia, are often acknowledged for advancing public participation, early bystander intervention, and high-quality implementation of CPR programs. In this sense, CPR became a shared effort across nations, rather than the achievement of any single nation. The formation of international partnerships, culminating in coordinated efforts including global guideline alignment in the 1990s, helped bring greater consistency to CPR practices worldwide.

As CPR spread across regions in the 1970s and 1980s, different countries developed their own training methods and guidelines, leading to variations in technique and practice. In response to these inconsistencies, the International Liaison Committee on Resuscitation (ILCOR) was formed in 1992. Uniting organizations from the United States, Europe, Canada, Australia, New Zealand, South Africa, and Latin America, ILCOR created a framework for a coordinated international approach to resuscitation science.

Rather than *replacing* national organizations, ILCOR concentrated on reviewing emerging research, building evidence-based consensus, and encouraging alignment of guidelines across regions. This collaboration led to greater international consistency, culminating in the 2000 International Guidelines for CPR and Emergency Cardiovascular Care, one of the first globally coordinated updates. Recurring review of processes and shared scientific evaluation helped standardize key elements such as compression rates, ventilation strategies, and AED use. Through this process, CPR evolved from a collection of national practices into a globally coordinated system of care. Training materials have been translated, adapted, and distributed across diverse populations, allowing CPR to become accessible internationally.

Concurrently, CPR guidelines were simplified to encourage broader participation. Emphasis on chest compressions, the introduction of Hands-Only CPR, and the integration of AED use made it easier for untrained bystanders to act quickly and confidently. These changes reduced hesitation and increased the likelihood of early bystander intervention.

CPR became a global public health movement because it was standardized, taught, practiced, and continuously refined across nations. CPR represents a unique intersection of science, education, and community action. It is one of the few medical interventions that relies as much on public participation as it does on professional care. Ultimately, CPR evolved into a global public health movement built on shared science, widespread training, and community action, not the work of any one country.

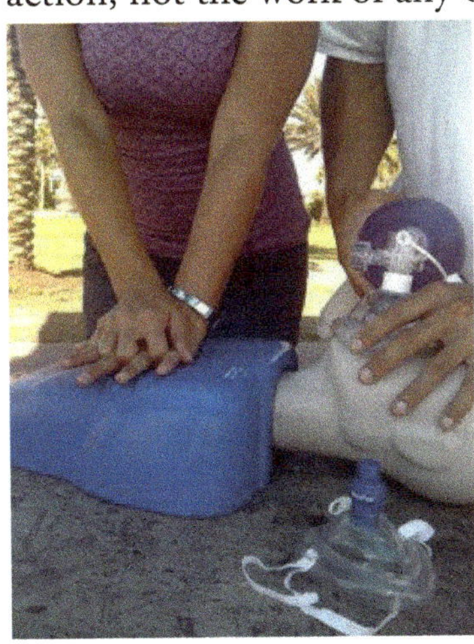

It was kind of at this point in time when I personally began to feel the rhythm of the CPR movement. When I first became a CPR instructor, Rescue Anne was becoming a less common CPR manikin, and I choose another, more lightweight manikin for my classes. One manikin line, the CPR Prompt manikin manufactured by Nasco, is near and dear to my heart because that was the first manikin I used to teach CPR classes. They were lightweight, easy to clean and assemble, and super affordable.

I was trying to figure out what to do with said manikins. With the advancements of technology, the CPR community really opened up for me. When I first started teaching CPR, my mother and I were pretty much the only CPR instruc-

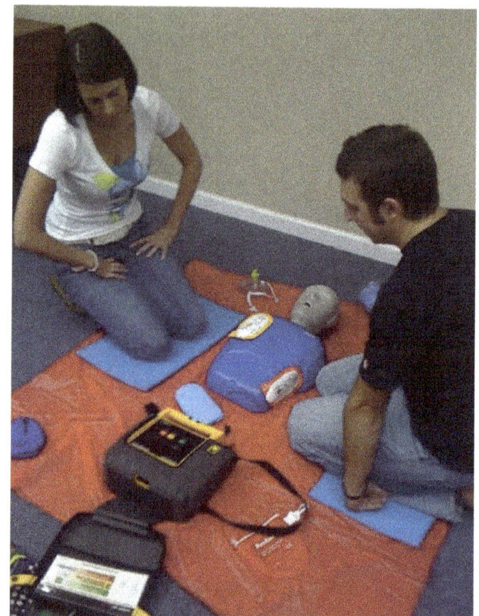

tors who I knew personally. Today, it seems like 1 in 20 healthcare providers is an instructor. (That is not in any way an exact number.) But now there are plenty of instructors, businesses, groups, and organizations where CPR advocates can commune. One such place is the CPR Instructor Network Facebook group. In 2025 in said group, I ran into Bob Kaplan, of Kaplan Sales & Marketing, as I was trying to figure out what to do with said manikins. I learned that plenty of people still use Prompt manikins.

In the mid-1990s Bob began working in a start-up in Solon, Ohio, called County Line Limited. The company was founded around 1992, and it later rebranded as CPR Prompt. The company introduced patented consumer products.

I appreciate Bob's perspective because he approached the CPR industry differently than many healthcare professionals. He viewed the field through the lenses of business, distribution, and market behavior, which gave him a unique perspective on how CPR products were developed, marketed, and sold.

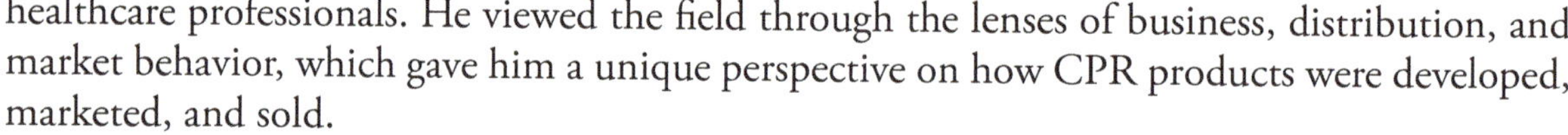

One of CPR Prompt's patented computer products was an early CPR guidance device called the CPR Prompt. It was a wall-mounted, voice guidance device that walked users through CPR steps—long before smart phones existed. Bob's perspective reflects a shift toward innovation within this space, when the focus moved from instruction alone to the creation and distribution of practical training products.

Later, the company created a CPR Prompt home learning system, including manikins and a VHS training tape endorsed by the AHA. The home learning system was sold in major retail stores, but it performed poorly, because back then consumers were not motivated to learn CPR.

"This was before the internet, before smartphones," Bob said. "This device would take you through the whole procedure of CPR. God forbid, you're in a situation where someone has sudden cardiac arrest. What are you going to do? Shoppers would just walk by. They wanted to look at that toaster oven. They didn't care about learning CPR."

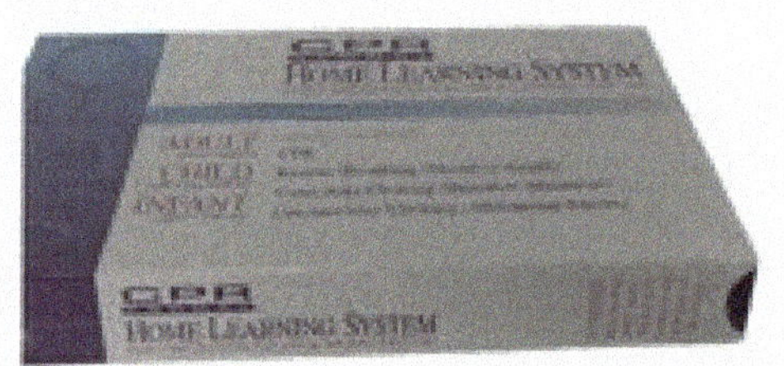

Those early devices laid the foundation for the development of many of the tools used in CPR education today.

Then the company pivoted, marketing their products to training centers and working with distributors like WorldPoint and Channing Bete. The original manikins were meant to be used in home, a few times a year, and weren't designed for an abundance of use. The engineers redesigned the manikins with more durable materials so they could be used by training centers.

Several other CPR training devices were developed, including handheld voice prompts, metronome trainers, and early universal AED trainers. Nasco conducted focus groups with EMS personnel, healthcare workers, and training centers to develop more advanced manikin designs. Just before these findings could be created and put into distribution, the company was sold to Cardiac Science, which focused primarily on AED sales. Bob went on to work for WorldPoint, distributing training equipment, and as the AHA regional manager for AHA training centers. He then managed an AHA training center of his own for 10 years in Seattle.

> The CPR Prompt would take you through the whole procedure of CPR. God forbid, you're in a situation where someone has sudden cardiac arrest. What are you going to do? Shoppers would just walk by. They wanted to look at that toaster oven. They didn't care about learning CPR.
> —Bob Kaplan

"Running a training center gave me the inside scoop on what people actually experience—the goods, the bads, and the challenges," Bob said.

Bob explained that early AED adoption was slow because people didn't really understand the devices, and businesses were fearful of liability.

"Back then, people looked at you like you had three ears when you said, 'Here's an AED,'" Bob said.

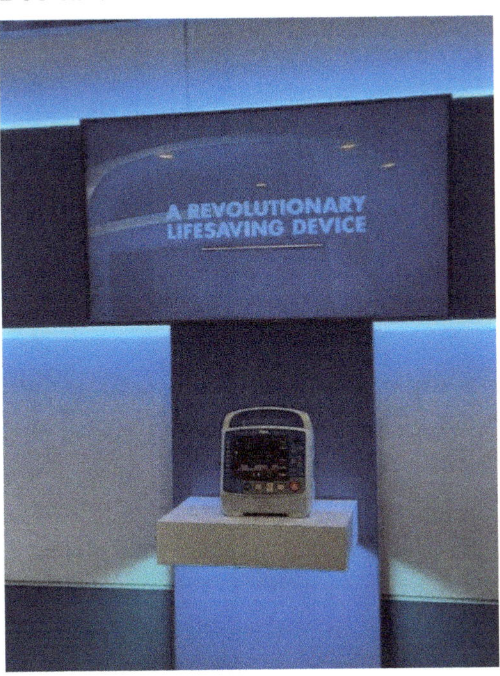

Bob expressed that PhysicControl dominated the AED market with their LifePak units into the 2000s. It was a major selling point that LifePak units were compatible with fire departments. One of my first AED trainers in the early days of People's Choice CPR was a LifePak.

Later, regulatory issues allowed competitors such as ZOLL, Philips, and Cardiac Science to expand their influence. Bob explained that AED sales became highly competitive and many CPR training businesses partnered with distributors instead of selling devices independently and directly to customers.

It is amazing to me how the CPR industry has turned into a major ecosystem of training equipment and AEDs over the years. When my mother and I first started People's Choice CPR, we valued always adding a little bit of *je ne sais quoi* by dressing our manikins to simulate real life and dramatically embellishing scenarios to encourage engagement. Today, so many tools and training pieces are available to add personal, realistic touches to CPR training.

About that training experience, who are we, these instructors? The instructors who disseminate CPR knowledge into classrooms, workplaces and communities across the globe are the rhythm keepers. We are a varied bunch.

For example, Jeffrey Gladney, one of my mentors, explained that he has been teaching for more than three decades. He got his first instructor certification in 1992. At first, he taught CPR classes occasionally, but then it became his full-time job. Then he expanded beyond CPR into first aid, universal precautions, drug testing, leadership development, and mentorship. Jeffrey brings skills and experience he gained from his military service and EMT training to all that he does. His work as a licensed minister and active church member also shapes his approach.

Scan to learn more about the Purpose Behind the Pulse with Jeffrey Gladney.

"Teaching is not only my passion. It's my purpose," Jeffrey said.

Another CPR instructor, my good friend, fellow author, and founder of Stress Free CPR, Renee Patterson, shared her passion and purpose about CPR with me. Renee is an EMT and 911 dispatcher, but her motivation for becoming a CPR instructor is more personal. When her son was little, she had left him with her mother, who called to say, "There's blood everywhere!" Renee understood that her mother called her rather than 911 because people often panic during potential emergencies.

Scan to learn more about Renee Patterson's story.

The best way to prevent panic is preparation. Accurate, engaging training prepares people to act when needed. "People need to know CPR," Renee said. "You never know what's going to happen when you walk out the door in the morning." Renee has written more than 12 children's books that teach children how to respond in emergencies.

> People need to know CPR. You never know what's going to happen when you walk out the door in the morning.
> — Renee Patterson, Founder of Stress Free CPR

My most memorable, inspiring CPR instructor story came from my favorite CPR instructor, Cia Sone-McClinton. In the early 1980s, Cia studied respiratory therapy, which required CPR training and laid the groundwork for her later becoming a CPR instructor. (I guess for all intents and purposes for me too!)

Cia came from a medically interested family. Her grandmother was a nurse who specialized in

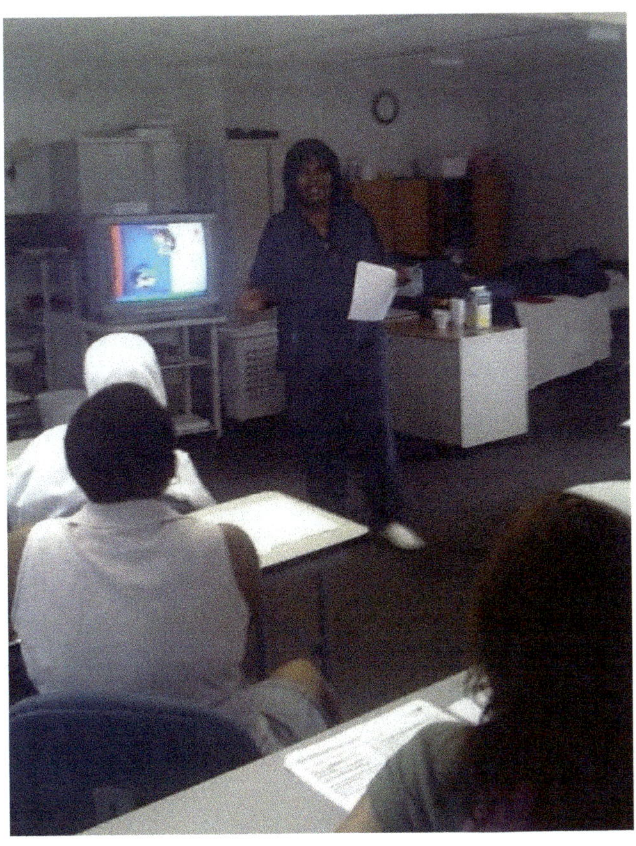

EKG monitoring, and her mother had worked in the surgery department in a Cleveland hospital. Cia finished her training and became a registered respiratory therapist.

As Cia's career progressed, she worked across intensive care units, coronary care units, emergency rooms, pediatric floors, and medical-surgical units. She experienced CPR not as a concept, but as a lived *reality*. She performed resuscitation on patients of every age—from the elderly to the impossibly small. One memory never left Cia: performing CPR on a neonate of 24 weeks.

"I could hold the baby in the palm of my hand, and I did CPR with just one finger, wondering if I was even going deep enough," Cia said.

Months later, that baby went home.

That moment didn't just reinforce the importance of CPR for Cia. It *defined* it. Cia didn't become an instructor because she had to. "I knew that CPR was something I could get behind and something valuable to know," Cia said. She truly appreciated the opportunity to interact with the community. "It was nice to teach not just healthcare professionals, but everyday people—expectant parents, babysitters, and anyone else who wanted to know how to do CPR."

Cia taught CPR through her hospital employment from the 1980s until 2009. It became even more personal for her when Michael Jackson died suddenly, reportedly from cardiac arrest. "If Michael Jackson could die from sudden cardiac arrest, I thought *Wow*," Cia said. That moment wasn't about celebrity. It was about vulnerability. It made cardiac arrest feel universal. And that was the turning point. Later that year, she made a decision.

> I could hold the baby in the palm of my hand, and I did CPR with just one finger, wondering if I was even going deep enough.
> —Cia Sone-McClinton, founder of People's Choice CPR.

Random fun fact, I often think of Michael Jackson when we ask during CPR, "Annie, are you okay?" as referenced in his song *Smooth Criminal*. Michael Jackson might have used the line "Annie, are you okay?" in that song because it captures the instinctive, real-life response to a person in distress.

Scan to learn More Than CPR with Cia Stone-McClinton of People's Choice CPR.

That phrase mirrors how people naturally check on a victim—especially in emergencies—by urgently asking if they are okay, which also aligns with the first step in CPR assessment.

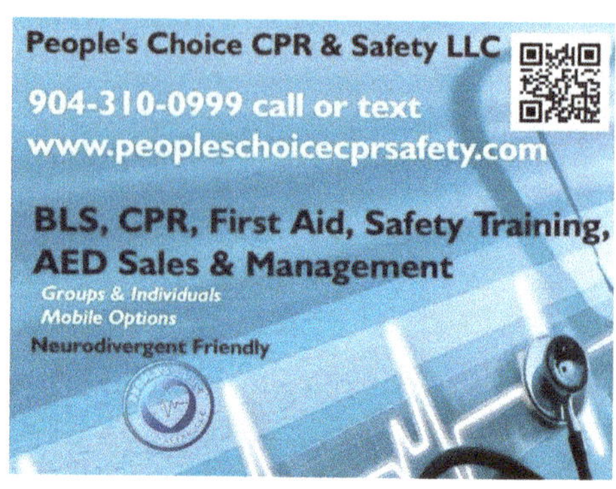

By using the name "Annie," the moment feels more personal and human, while the repetition of the line builds tension and reinforces the seriousness of the situation. At the same time, the phrasing fits the rhythm of the song perfectly, making it both emotionally impactful and musically memorable.

Anyway, Cia decided she would build something of her own. She had always wanted to start a business, and she realized that CPR empowered people to help others when they needed it most. People's Choice CPR was born in September 2009.

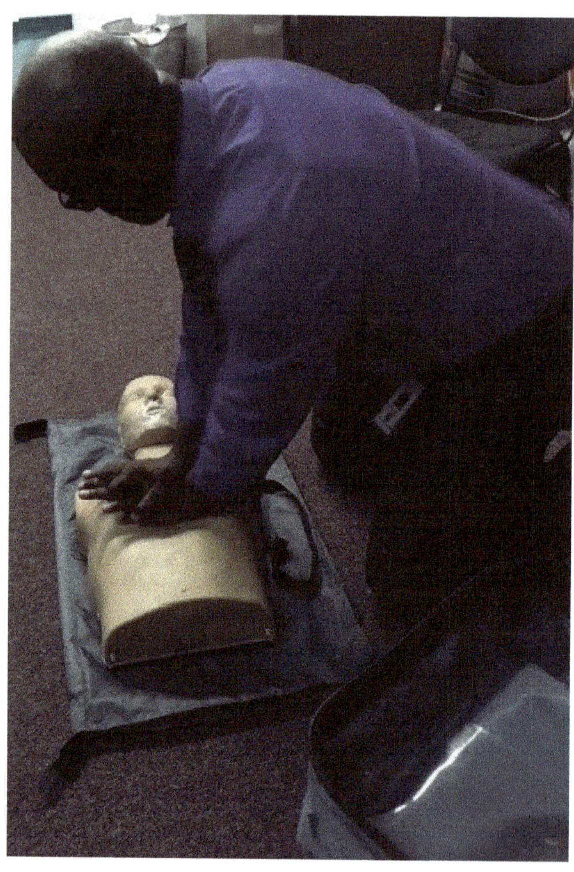

Chapter 7: A Movement with a Pulse

Scan to learn more about MCR Medical.

Now, we had instructors teaching classes, but we needed training *supplies*: manikins, manikin lung bags, face shields, pocket masks, bag-mask devices, and more! Particular equipment is required for certain classes. Not having the proper equipment can put an instructor or program out of compliance. It can also contribute to class disengagement.

I've been known to live by the seat of my pants. At times, I've definitely cut some things close, especially in my early days. But I could always count on MCR Medical to quickly get me together.

My mother came to know MCR Medical through Karen Morrison, the company's cofounder. Back then, my mother and I lived so close to Karen that rather than mailing supplies to us, we would pick them up from Karen's mailbox, or she would drop them off in ours. I loved how quickly MCR Medical grew because they could ship to Florida, which was helpful to me because in 2010, I went on vacation there—and never left.

Fast forward to 2023. My mother and I ran into Wes Almond, Vice President and Chief Operating Officer of MCR Medical, at my beloved Lifesaving Summit. (More on that in Chapter 9.) MCR Medical is a proud continual sponsor of the Lifesaving Summit, which shows their commitment to staying in sync with instructors. I have to say Wes is a great company representative because he is so genuine, truly a likable, funny individual. It totally made sense that he had become part of MCR Medical. We were delighted to be reacquainted with MCR Medical in a new way. Hanging out with Wes, and later the entire MCR Medical team, is always a delight.

> There's nothing worse than having a training scheduled for tomorrow, and you don't have your supplies yet.
> —Wes Almond, Vice President and Chief Operating Officer of MCR Medical

Recently, (admittedly, that is relative to when you're reading this book), I had the opportunity to interview Wes for an episode of the Wellness Pulse celebrating National CPR Week 2025. I wanted to share about the history of MCR Medical, their growth, and their close relationship with instructors. I wanted to shine a light on how MCR Medical's impact extends beyond manufacturing products into community initiatives, workforce inclusion, and advancing CPR training through technology.

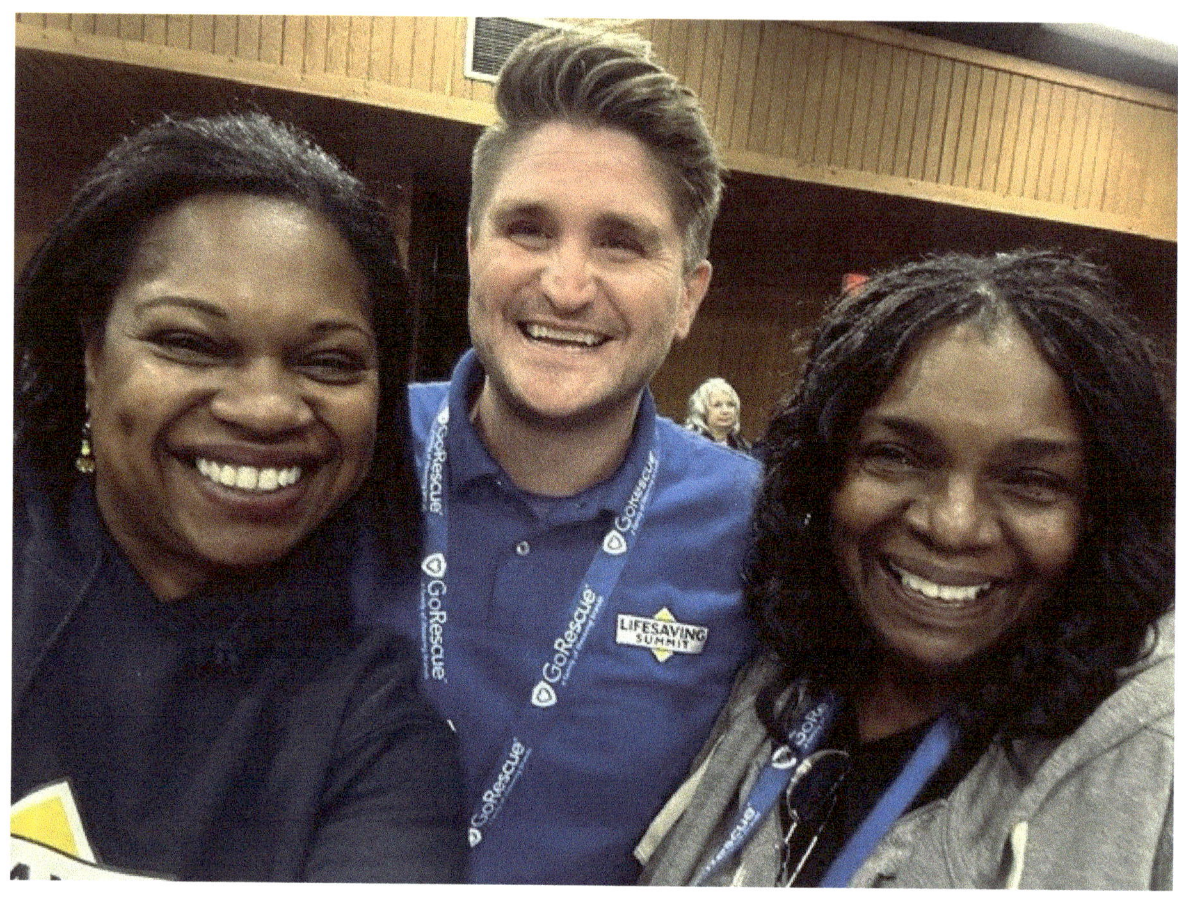

MCR Medical is a hybrid manufacturer and distributor of CPR and first aid supplies. They are the bridge between CPR manufacturers and instructors.

Built on service, relationships, and purpose-driven distribution, the company focuses on equipping educators with reliable, high-quality tools while innovating based on real-world feedback. MCR actively gathers feedback from instructors through events and relationships, then works with engineers and product teams to create solutions that address real classroom challenges.

MCR Medical's products, including manikins, clothing, AED kits, and engagement tools like the clothing for the manikins or disposable cardboard scissors for simulation with AED or first aid training, are designed to make training realistic, memorable, and effective. Their innovation is driven by real instructor needs.

"We really have to strategize on how we can connect with our customer base. We can learn from them and get a better understanding of what their pain points are," Wes said.

MCR Medical collaborates with manufacturers, such as PRESTAN. They closely adhere to industry standards, such as American Heart Association (AHA) guidelines, ensuring quality, consistency, and effectiveness in training tools. Wes emphasized that careful partner selection, quality assurance, and reliability are critical to avoiding supply failures that could disrupt training.

In our interview, Wes stated that the heart of MCR Medical centers on PRESTAN training manikins and the consumable products that support CPR instructors and training centers, including manikin, lung bags, replacement parts, face shields, one way valves, and first aid training supplies.

For as long as I can recall, MCR Medical has been the premier distributor for PRESTAN. Wes stated that "their bread and butter," centers on Prestan training manikins and the consumable products that support CPR instructors and training centers.

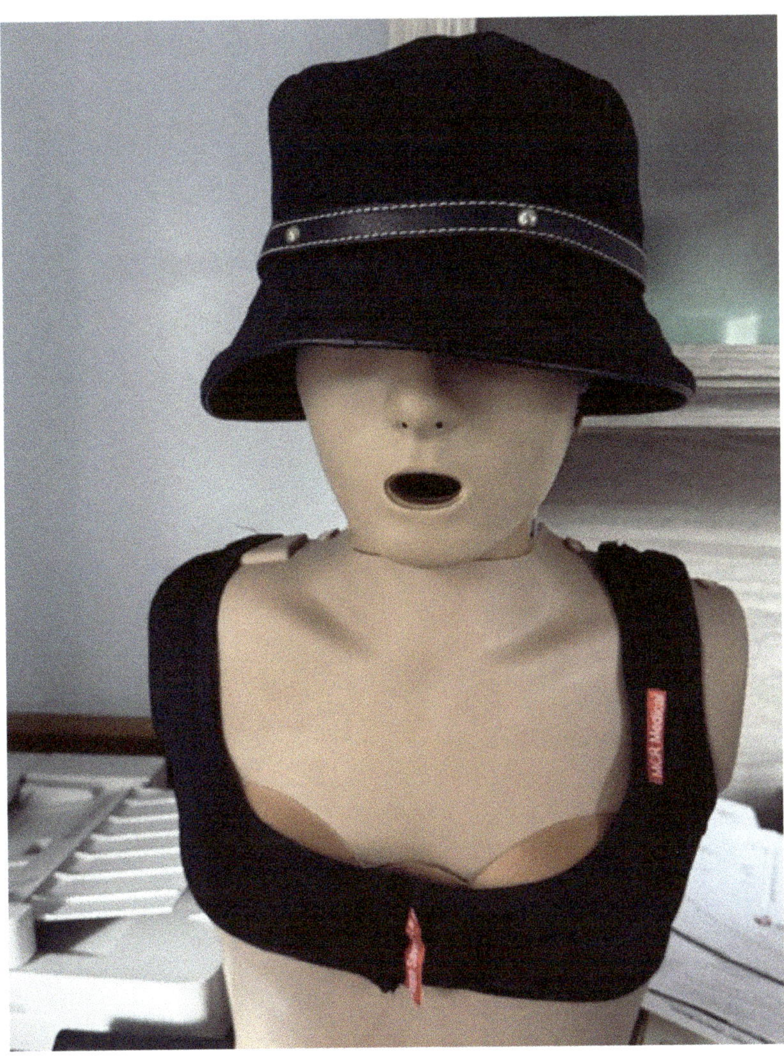

That brings me back to Karen Morrison, who aggressively petitioned PRESTAN to distribute PRESTAN manikins and training supplies. Even though MCR Medical was not the ideal distributor at that time, the rest is history, as they say! Karen wanted instructors to have realistic, high-quality manikins that she could believe in. As a result, there's clothing for the manikins!

"It's not every day you're going to walk up on a patient, and they're going to be naked," Wes joked.

In our interview, he described how MCR Medical began in 2008 in Columbus, Ohio, when Charlie and Karen Morrison started the business in a spare bedroom during the economic downturn. Both faced shrinking incomes, Charlie in a family-owned business and Karen in the mortgage industry. The couple listed their strengths and passions, and they identified a gap in the CPR and first-aid training supply market. Drawing on volunteer experience and a shared passion for helping people, they launched a small distribution business just as e-commerce was beginning to blossom. The company steadily grew. Then in 2012, bursting out of their garage and spare bedroom, they purchased their first warehouse.

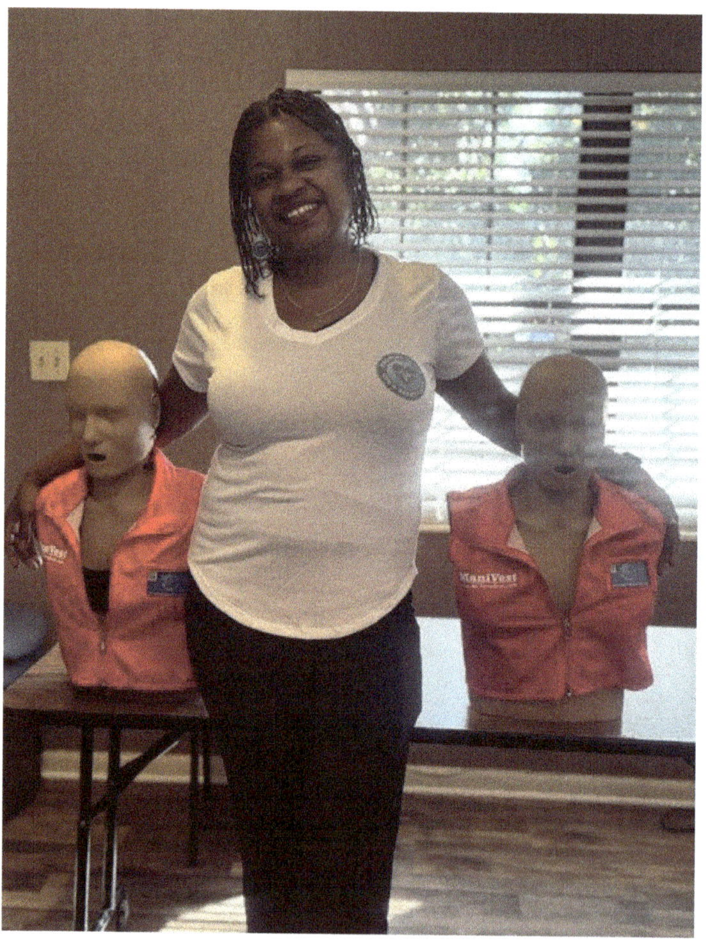

Wes explained how the company's growth accelerated once they committed full-time to MCR Medical. At that point, the team consisted of just Charlie, Karen, and one other employee.

To expand their workforce, Charlie and Karen joined the Columbus Chamber of Commerce, where they met Wes. He brought deep experience in employing adults with disabilities, having previously managed programs that placed hundreds of people in meaningful jobs across many industries. Wes's background aligned perfectly with the founders' values, and soon Wes became part of the MCR Medical family. His commitment to creating opportunities for people of all abilities became a cornerstone of the company's culture.

Wes expressed pride in this inclusive approach, noting that people from all walks of life contributed to the business's success. "We're actual humans behind this operation, and we care," he said. A guiding principle of the company is treating *all* people with care and dignity.

Wes shared stories of exceptional customer service during the company's early days. Before their warehouse was fully operational, Charlie and Karen often delivered products directly to customers' doorsteps or mailboxes. Instructors never lacked equipment for classes, even if they were living by the seat of their pants and ordering with very little time to spare, like me.

I shared with Wes how my journey as a CPR instructor intertwined with MCR Medical's evolution. I remembered purchasing early PRESTAN manikins through MCR Medical. Encounters with MCR Medical staff at lifesaving conferences over the years reinforced my admiration for the team's dedication and warmth.

Every visit to MCR Medical revealed a workplace full of energy and genuine happiness. I visit MCR Medical whenever I am in Columbus, Ohio, which could be once or a few times each year. They might not get a lot of consumers visiting their warehouse because they are an online distributor, but through our connection at the Lifesaving Summit, they invited me to tour the warehouse. I took them up on it. Now, I visit regularly.

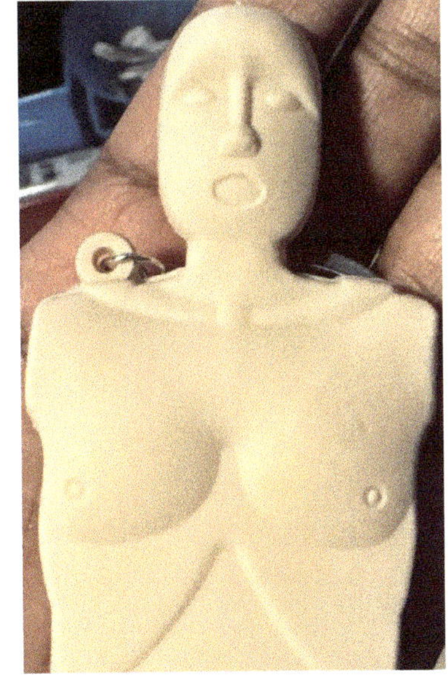

I think it's cool to know the engineers and staff behind the products. How often does that happen? Do you personally know the person who made your purse or undergarments? I admire MCR Medical's focus on work-life balance and the respect they show to every employee. If *I* lived in Columbus, I would definitely work there. I love how MCR Medical has grown from a spare-bedroom startup to an internationally recognized supplier, while keeping their heart for service that first attracted my family as customers.

As pick-me-ups and incentives for CPR instructors, MCR Medical offers a lot of cool, non-traditional, innovative items, including PRESTAN manikin keychains, rolling bags, instructor customized manikin kits, and much more. Wes described how these inexpensive but thoughtful trinkets help students remember their training and gave them positive feelings about CPR.

MCR Medical offers innovative items for their employees as well. Buckets of fidget toys and tubs of Play-Doh spark creativity during meetings. As a fellow educator, I appreciate these details and how MCR Medical takes such care to foster a vibrant culture that keeps employees inspired. Wes emphasized that these touches are more than fun. They are part of a broader philosophy, a touchstone "What would Karen Morrison do?" Karen's focus on treating every person with respect shaped their approach to employees and customers alike.

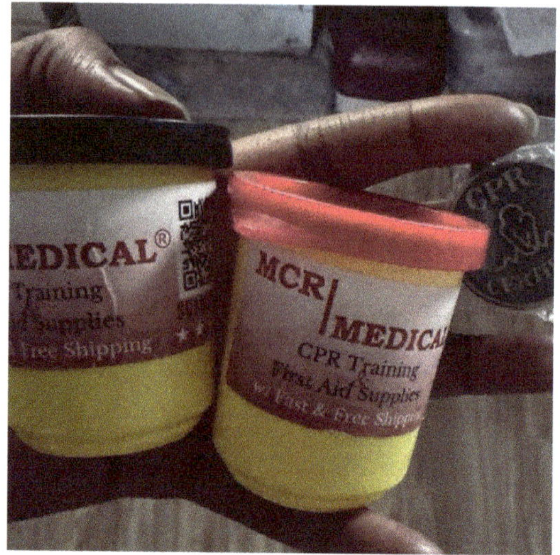

That dedication has shown in every interaction I have had with the company. MCR Medical's consistent growth brought both recognition and responsibility. The company earned a spot on the Columbus Business First Fast 50 list for ten consecutive years, a testament to its rapid expansion. Wes himself was named to the city's list of 40 Under 40. The company and its leaders have received multiple Diversity Champion awards. Also, Charlie Morrisson was honored as Small Business Leader of the Year by the Columbus Chamber of Commerce.

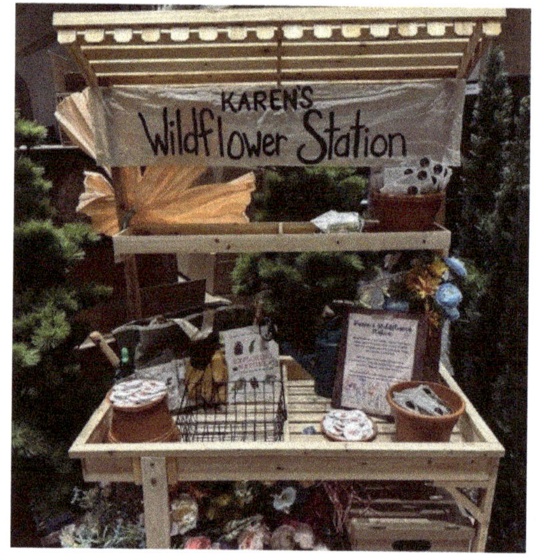

Personally, I feel this public recognition mirrors the private culture I have experienced. MCR Medical is rooted in service, respect, and community impact. I admire and appreciate their ongoing commitment to giving back to communities.

For example, they support literacy programs through local libraries, contribute to homeless outreach efforts, support initiatives for women entrepreneurs, and continue to create job opportunities for people of all abilities, integrating social impact into their business model. I love MCR Medical's heart for helping people, employees, customers, instructors, and community members alike.

Scan to check out day 1 of the CASS 2025.

Chapter 8: The Bias in the Beat

Scan to learn more about PRESTAN.

I fondly remember the feeling of upgrading to my first PRESTAN manikin. It is hard to describe in words. What comes close is the old expression, "You couldn't tell me nothing," or a feeling of pride and exhilaration. I knew that I could use the new manikins to deliver high-quality skills to teach effectively memorable classes.

Since then, I've taught many classes at a ocean-front park using PRESTAN products, and I will always associate them with a life upgrade. PRESTAN makes more realistic manikins, with lights in the shoulder that visually communicate to students if they are reaching the right depth and the right rate for high-quality compressions. PRESTAN manikins also feature a clicker in the chest to assist with fostering muscle memory, identifying what it feels like to reach the appropriate depth for adequate compressions. These manikins definitely increased my confidence as an instructor because I knew that the students who took my classes would build confidence from the skills acquired from using these high-quality manikins.

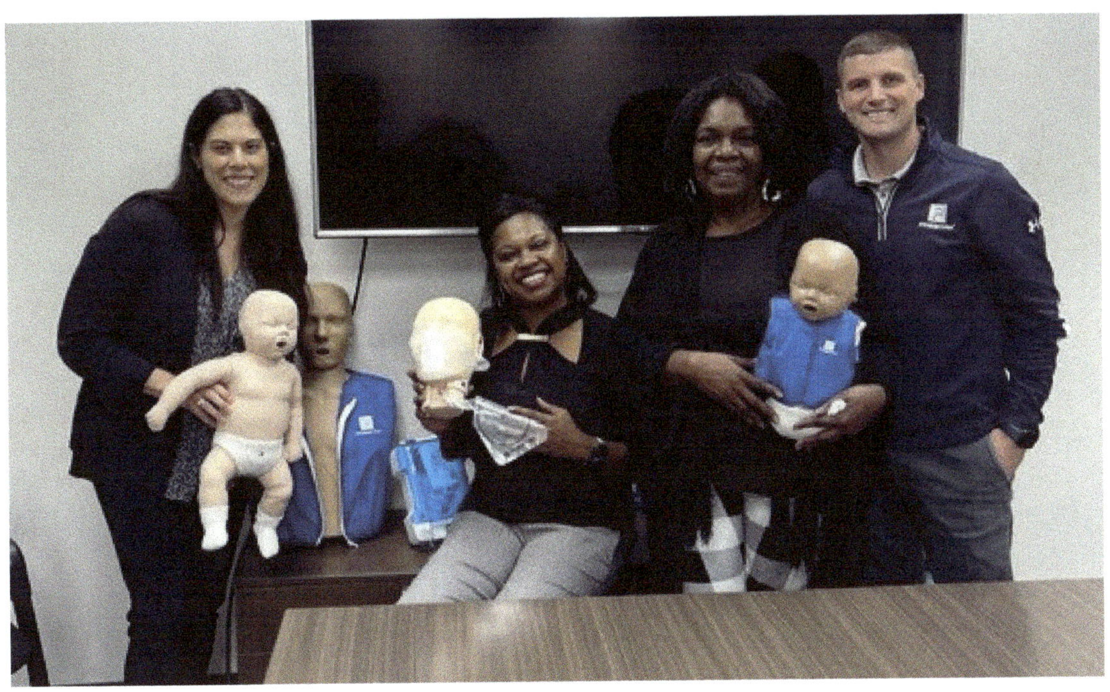

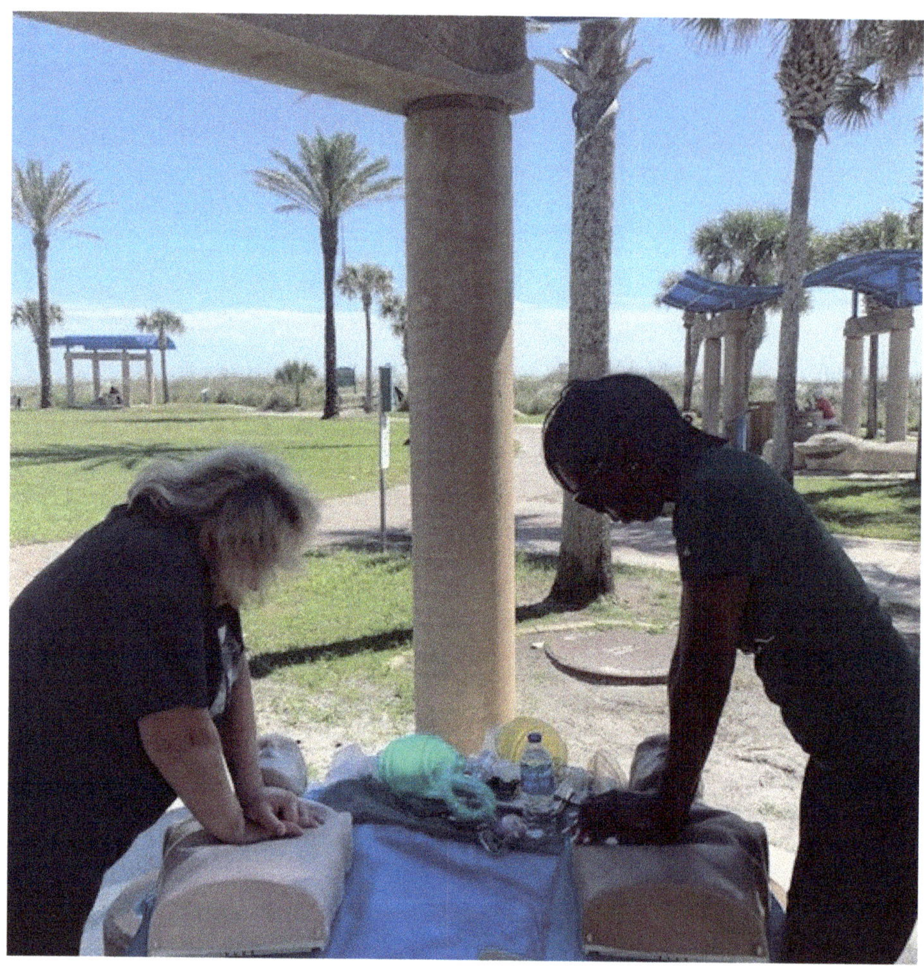

At the 2023 Lifesaving Summit in Birmingham, Alabama, I participated in a PRESTAN focus group. (More on my beloved Lifesaving Summit in Chapter 9.) I was very excited. How often do you get to ask questions about and offer input on products you use? The PRESTAN staff was wonderful! Cory and Lindsay showed me such a great time and showed me products, including the Professional Manikin Plus, a prototype of the Professional Manikin Plus head, and the female breast attachment that preceded the female manikin skin.

Through conversations with PRESTAN team members at the Lifesaving Summit and beyond, I have become even more impressed with PRESTAN. They consistently support instructors like me, and they produce durable, high-quality manikins and accessories.

PRESTAN was founded in 2004 near Cleveland, Ohio, and is committed to providing CPR training manikins and AED trainers that are intuitive, durable, cost-effective, and designed to build confidence through immediate feedback. Since then, PRESTAN has grown from a small start-up funded by three founders and four small investors to a global company serving customers in more than eighty countries with warehousing and distribution worldwide.

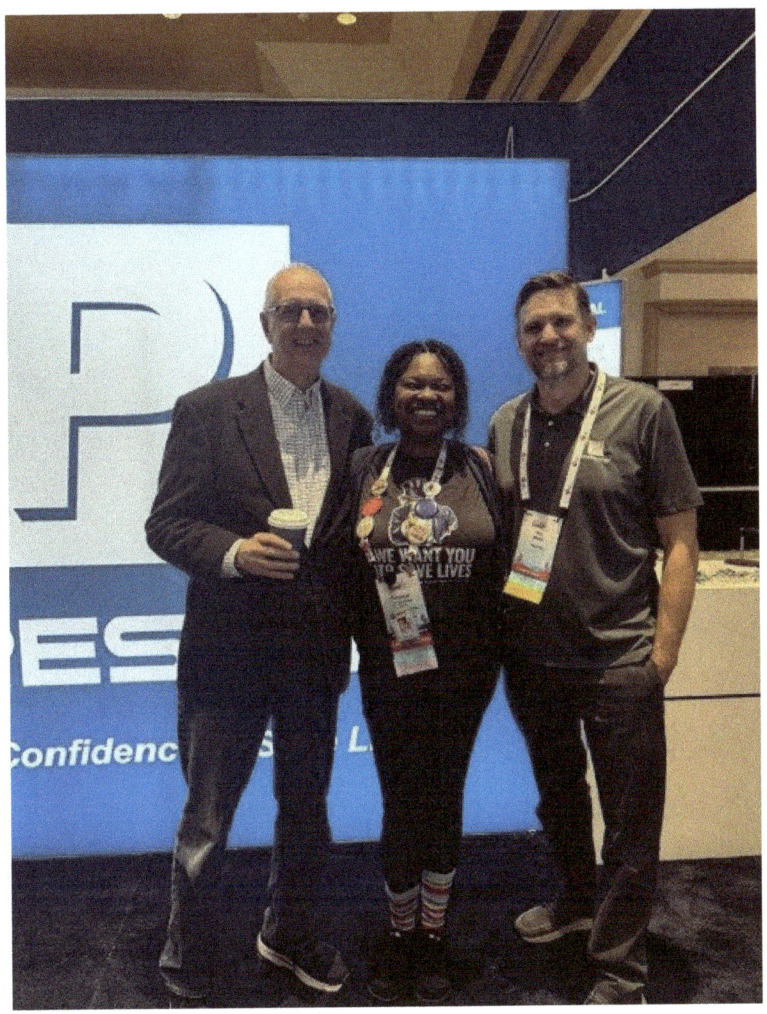

I recently had the chance to talk with Lindsay Benz, Director of Global Marketing of PRESTAN, for my podcast, the Wellness Pulse. Lindsay supports PRESTAN's distribution network while also connecting with instructors, nonprofits, end users like CPR instructors, and industry organizations like the American Heart Association and ILCOR. Because PRESTAN sells through distributors such as MCR Medical rather than directly to instructors, those client relationships are essential.

PRESTAN is actively involved in industry events, including the Cardiac Arrest Survival Summit, the Lifesaving Summit, Parent Heart Watch, and the National CPR and AED Rally and March. These events and vice versa give the company the opportunity to interact with the end users of their products. PRESTAN is often two or three steps removed from instructors who are actually using their products in classes. The events are opportunities to hold focus groups, hear what instructors like and dislike, and identify needs where the company can add value.

PRESTAN's design philosophy is simple: Everything revolves around building confidence. They make CPR training equipment, but their ultimate goal is to help students and instructors feel prepared to perform CPR.

Lindsay shared that PRESTAN's team spent time early on understanding how adults learn. One major insight was that adults do not like being publicly called out for doing something wrong. That creates anxiety and discomfort. That's why PRESTAN designed their manikins to be intuitive and self-correcting. The lights in the shoulder and the click in the chest support intuition and self-correction ability. A student can watch for the lights and listen for the click and adjust if necessary—without being singled out by the instructor.

Mode	Light 1	Light 2	Light 3	Light 4
Sleep Mode/No Power	○	○	○	○
1st Full Compression (Wake mode/LED Test Mode)	● (green)	● (red)	● (yellow)	● (green)
CPM* < 60	○	● (red)	○	○
CPM* 60 – 79	○	○	● (yellow)	○
CPM* 80 – 99	● (green)	○	○	○
CPM* 100 - 120	● (green)	○	○	● (green)
CPM* > 120	● (green)	○	● (yellow, flashing)	● (green)
Compressions Stopped	○	● (red, flashing)	○	○

*CPM = Compressions per minute
= Flashing

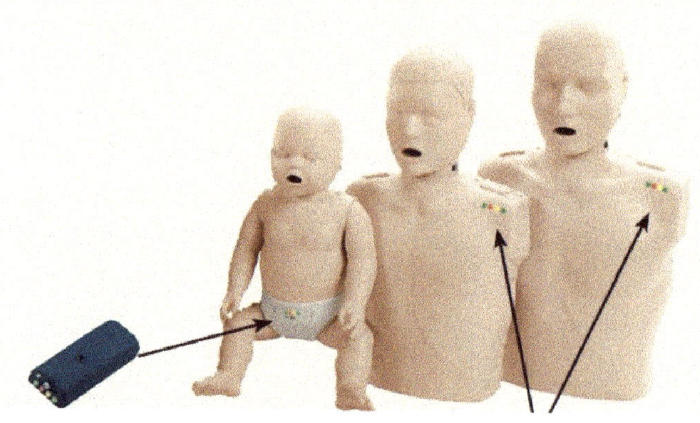

"Instructors are not just consumers, they are co-creators," Lindsay said. "PRESTAN listens to instructors to refine tools, close gaps, and keep pushing CPR education toward realism, usability, and confidence."

Once students begin seeing the lights and feeling the compression depth, it quickly becomes muscle memory. Lindsay recalled watching nervous school staff move from uncertainty to real confidence in a short period of time. I can definitely attest to the same phenomenon.

Lindsay explained that PRESTAN eventually moved beyond the original, gray-skinned manikins and introduced medium- and dark-skin options, as well as diversity manikin kits that feature both skin tones in one instructor kit, so classrooms could better reflect the population. She recommends instructors strive for realistic representation, using male and female manikins with different skin tones and of different ages. If students only train on one type of manikin, they may be more likely to hesitate in any real-life situation that looks different from their training. PRESTAN offers a family or group of manikins, and purchasers can elect to have them shipped in one skin tone or various configurations.

Professional Female Manikin

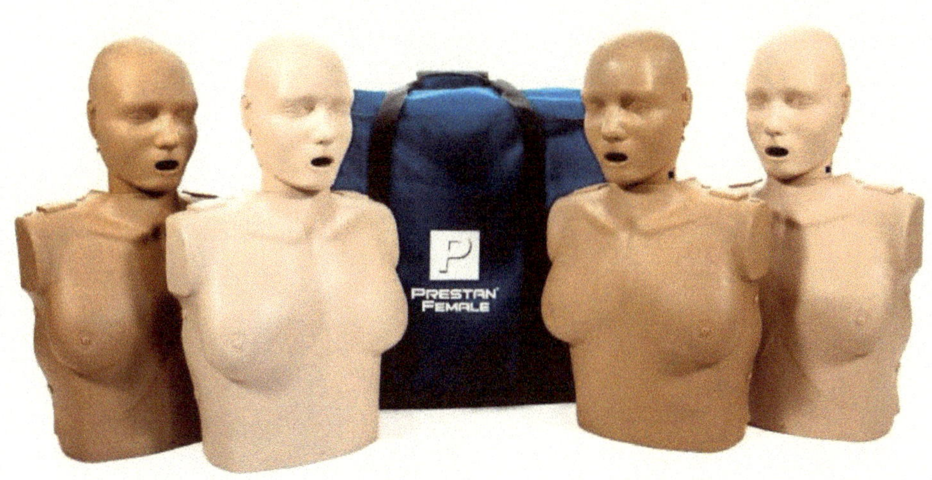

I know some people disagree and don't value details like that. But gender matters. Even when cardiac arrest is witnessed in public, women receive bystander CPR less often than men—39 percent compared to 45 percent, according to a 2018 study published in *Circulation* by Audrey L. Blewer and colleagues. Drawing on data from the Resuscitation Outcomes Consortium, the study revealed a measurable and consequential gender disparity in early resuscitation—one that persists despite widespread CPR education and has direct implications for survival.

On the day that I wrote this chapter, I had a gentleman in my class uncomfortable with the female manikin. He repeatedly covered the breast and was reluctant to interact with the nipple. It was comical, but it was a private class, and he wasn't embarrassed when I chuckled.

It was a magnificent teaching opportunity! My lady manikin was wearing an MCR Medical Mani-Bra and a PRESTAN jacket. The gentleman was able to get the full experience of undressing a woman to perform CPR. I shared a gender disparity statistic with him, along with my little saying, "Boobs usually get you *into* places, not *out of* places!" In that case, I mean out of life.

Lindsay said that CPR classrooms traditionally trained on male manikin torsos. As a result, many students never practiced removing a bra, moving breast tissue to place pads, or even touching a female chest out of fear or hesitation. As an instructor, I can attest that this has been true for me as well, but we *can* train students to be comfortable with performing CPR on manikins of both sexes moving forward.

Other advocates of this concept include the ladies of HeartCharged, a nonprofit organization founded by sisters Bethany Keime and Hannah Keime who both have hypertrophic cardiomyopathy and are focused on awareness and sudden cardiac arrest prevention, and Aubi Nehmeth, a CRNA in cardiac anesthesia and CPR instructor. These are a few of the advocates I have been personally inspired by. Their diligence in educating the world on these disparities and why inclusive teaching of CPR is a necessity. It's almost like history repeating itself, a lone outlier group championing a huge undertaking because it can save lives.

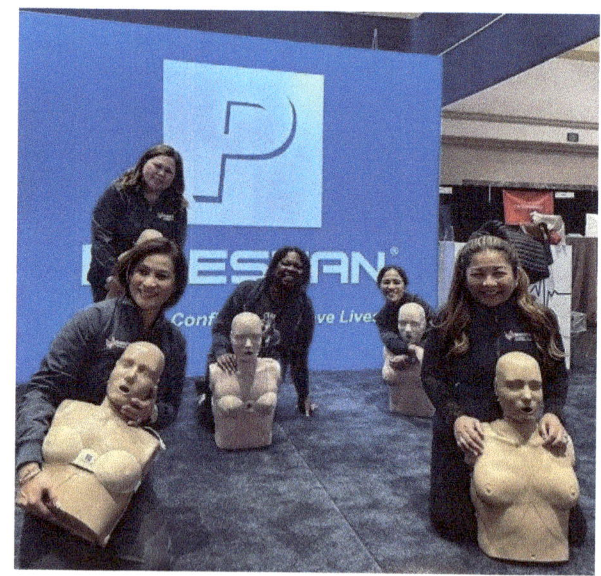

"Breasts do not change CPR, but they do change behavior," Aubi said.

Nothing changes mechanically, but behavior does, and because of that, women receive less CPR. People are afraid of being accused of inappropriate touching or assault. The fear of accusation is greater than the fear of doing nothing. People are more afraid of getting in trouble than of someone dying. They feel awkward, they don't know where to place their hands, and they worry about touching the wrong area—even on a manikin. If people hesitate on a manikin, what do we think will happen in real life?

"Bodies with breasts are not part of training," Aubi continued. "Ninety-five percent of CPR manikins are flat-chested, and even in a room full of instructors, only a minority have trained on a manikin with breasts. This is not sexual. It's not social. It's anatomy. We are making it an issue when it does not need to be."

"How does a lump of tissue stop you from saving a life?" Bethany asked. "That's somebody's life. You're going to be held accountable for letting her pass away because you didn't want to do what was right."

Scan to learn more about manikins with breasts.

Lindsay explained that PRESTAN created their female line to help participants get over the shock, fear, and hesitation in the classroom so people will not freeze during an emergency if the victim is a woman. She stated that because men are more likely to receive bystander CPR, they have a 23 percent higher chance of survival.

"This is unacceptable and tied directly to what people were, and were not, being exposed to in training," Lindsay said. "The answer is not to avoid the issue, but to talk it through in training. Learners need exposure before an emergency happens."

She is absolutely correct. Over the years, I've grown as an instructor and become more aware of how cultural, gender, and sexuality-related discomfort can interfere with action. Before I had female manikins, I used to describe the need to move large breasts out of the way to perform CPR. But the actual opportunity to use female manikins and allow students to do compressions and understand female anatomy in class is magnificent. In almost every class, I discover at least one student who understands why someone might hesitate to perform CPR on a woman. That's why I bring the female manikin to each of my classes.

PRESTAN's product line also expanded to include infant and child manikins, the Ultralite line, a lighter more portable PRESTAN manikin option, the female accessory, a clipable manikin breast attachment, and then full female manikin, the Series 2000 line with app-based advanced feedback on detailed CPR metrics of compression depth, rate, recoil and ventilation allowing for objective performance tracking, the Pro+ head with expanded nasal passage, which some instructors can use for advanced emergency skill classes like ACLS or even Narcan training, automated external defibrillator or AED trainers.

Many people still wrongly assume only medical professionals can use AEDs, so training tools must help demystify the devices. Students are comforted to learn that AEDs are built to guide ordinary people, not just professionals. I used to be surprised at how many people were unaware of AEDs. I like to show more than one AED style in my classes because real devices vary.

Lindsay explained PRESTAN's AED trainers were designed to reduce intimidation. She shared some insights on PRESTAN's Ultralite line, which was designed for community awareness events, independent instructors, portability, and affordability. These manikins are lightweight, and they disassemble. They are also less expensive than the other PRESTAN manikins.

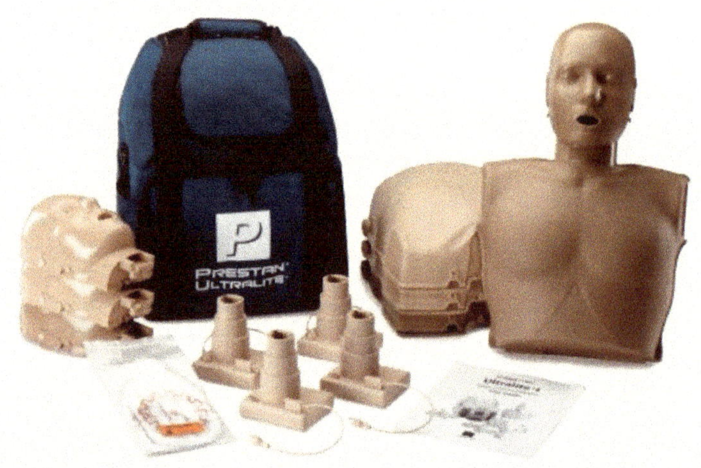

PORTABLE

Ultralite® Manikin Diversity Kits

They became popular for remote training during COVID. Because the Ultralite manikins pack compactly and are easier to ship, many instructors were able to keep teaching by mailing them to students and coaching through video calls.

PRESTAN's series 2000 line builds on the professional platform by integrating Bluetooth-enabled app-based advanced feedback. During classes, participants use the PRESTAN Series 2000 manikin, which provides real-time performance data and analytics—including recoil, hands-off time, ventilation feedback, and chest compression fraction, which are key indicators of high-quality CPR. This expanded data provides students and instructors with objective performance metrics and reporting, advancing CPR training from basic skill practice to measurable, high-quality resuscitation performance.

Although not every instructor chooses to switch entirely to that system, many use one or two series 2000 manikins in the classroom so students can see deeper metrics and understand where their compressions need refinement. Lindsay emphasized that recoil of a patient's chest matters because if the patient's chest does not fully release, blood flow is compromised. The visual data helps students understand what they *think* they are doing versus what they are *actually* doing.

Another innovative PRESTAN product, their newer Pro+ head, was originally developed for Germany, where breaths are delivered over the nose. Different countries have different

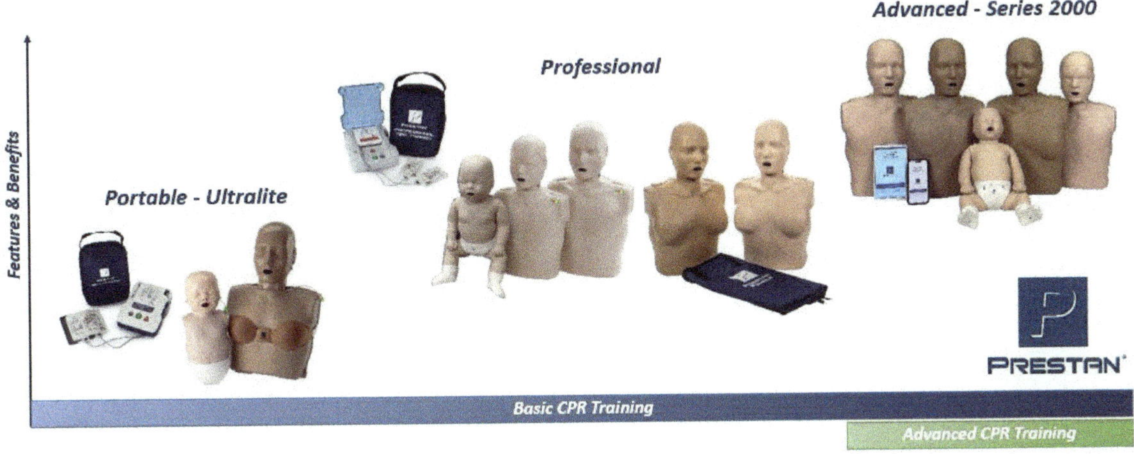

guidelines because each country is free to interpret resuscitation science. When the Pro+ head entered the market, instructors and trainers in the United States found additional uses for it, including Narcan training, Nasopharyngeal Airway (NPA) training, and Oropharyngeal Airway (OPA) practice. A nasopharyngeal airway (NPA) is inserted through the nose into the nasopharynx, whereas an oropharyngeal airway (OPA) is placed through the mouth into the oropharynx, each providing a pathway to maintain a patient's airway.

"This is a perfect example of why PRESTAN has to stay in constant conversation with the field," Lindsay said. "People often use products in ways the company did not initially predict."

I've also seen how PRESTAN respects instructors' investments in their products. For example, whenever possible, new features are designed as upgrades to existing manikins, rather than forcing instructors to replace entire manikins. Manikin replacement parts are available for instructors to repair or upgrade their stock.

Another important practice is designing their products for long-term classroom use. This matters because instructors like me carry, store, repair, clean, and transport these tools constantly.

PRESTAN's CPR training manikins are made in the United States. Lindsay said that this helps reduce supply delays and gives distributors more confidence in product availability.

Along with PRESTAN, I'm a CPR crusader. Together, we spread CPR love all over. It takes an entire village to make this work. It's so refreshing to be able to work with other people to advocate and educate. I bet many people didn't know that this much thought went into their CPR class.

Chapter 9: The Evolution of the Rhythm

At this point, I have mentioned the Lifesaving Summit (LSS) umpteenth times, without actually telling you what it is. I hold out no longer.

Scan to learn more about the Lifesaving Summit.

The LSS is what Miranda Burnette, leader of training and education at GoRescue, refers to as *CPR Christmas!* It's a fabulous time of year where CPR crusaders gather to collaborate, educate, learn, and build relationships. I would say *network,* but it is so much more than that. The LSS is typically held in October, in Alabama. I say typically, because in 2025, it was on a cruise that went to the Bahamas, in November!

Miranda herself shared with me that, "CPR is very close to my heart because I want to remember my why of why I started. On September 12, 2008, I lost my mother-in-law to sudden cardiac arrest. Knowing that training is available for a loved one to go home to their family is extremely important to me."

In 2023, the first year that my mother and I attended the Lifesaving Summit, I was impressed with all of the knowledge and ideas all in one room. Plus, all of these businesses, mostly entrepreneurs, are down-to-earth, kind people (or at least on their best behavior) and all super stoked about CPR and getting it out to the masses.

Scan to learn more about Miranda Burnette's story.

Because of the entrepreneurial spirit, all different flavors and kinds of business models are showcased at the LSS. We don't compete or sell while there. Instead, we team build and impart inspiration and ideas to each other. We form friendships that are like family, the kind of family you want to do business with, because they assist with business growth in ways sometimes rooted in personal growth. There is something for every stage of business at the LSS.

I was fortunate enough to chat with Brady McLaughlin, CEO and Founder of GoRescue, although he described himself as the chief firefighter and said, "My job is to put out fires, solve problems, and reduce friction so we can fulfill on our motto, which is lifesaving made easy for our clients. Every day, my job is to pour into our team so that our team can pour into our clients and students across the country, so that we can strengthen the chain of survival."

Brady shared how his company began. "In 2012, God gave me a very clear vision while my wife and I were sitting at our table. We were six months married and never wanted to have

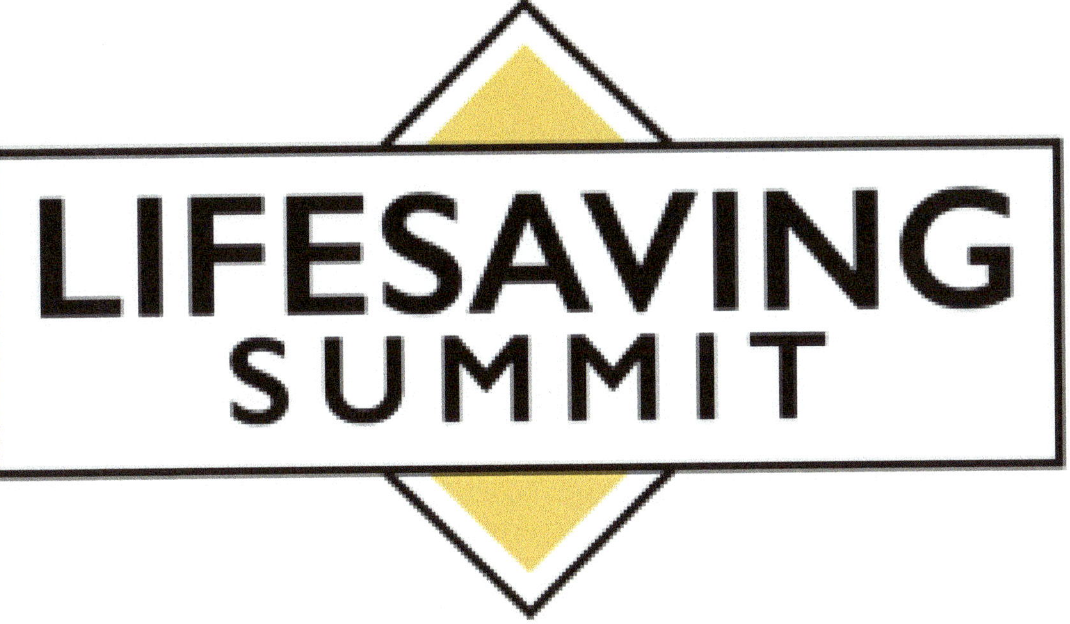

a business. The vision was clear: How do you save more lives outside the context of working a 12- or 24-hour shift? The answer was by training and equipping people. So we started an organization called TrioSafety."

During our interview, Brady explained that TrioSafety was the original CPR training company he founded to train and equip people in CPR and AED use. TrioSafety focused on providing hands-on lifesaving education while he continued working in public safety roles to support its growth without debt. Over time, as the business expanded and identified additional needs in the industry, Trio Safety merged with an AED-focused company (Stop Heart Attack), which ultimately contributed to the evolution and rebranding into what is now GoRescue—a more comprehensive organization offering training, equipment, and program management solutions across the lifesaving space.

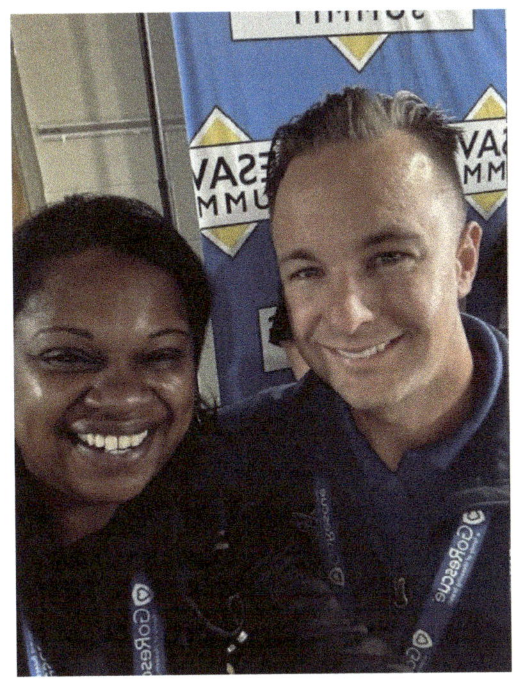

Brady has always had a passion for saving lives. In his early teens, he rode his bike to fire calls near his home. When he grew up, he became an EMT, volunteer firefighter, EMS dispatcher, police officer, then a paid firefighter. Even after he and his wife founded GoRescue, he continued to work in public safety as they built the business to bootstrap it and reinvest without taking on business debt.

One of many things I have learned from Brady is the power of collaboration. In 2017, TrioSafety made a local connection with Stop Heart Attack, an established AED-focused company. Founded in 1997, Stop Heart Attack's core strength was providing automated external defibrillators (AEDs) and related accessories. The two merged and became GoRescue. Then in 2024, GoRescue united with Safe Life, a private holding company that unites CPR training, AED distribution, and program management businesses to expand their reach and strengthen their collective impact all over the world. By connecting these services, it helps create a more complete lifesaving system, from training individuals to equipping environments and maintaining readiness over time.

Brady and his wife, Malynda, definitely supersized their dream of helping save more lives. Yet GoRescue is not content. "We also have a clear, 10-year target to deliver 1 million lifesaving impacts. For us, that means a student trained, an AED placed, an AED put on program management, or a bleeding control kit installed. We believe that after 10 years, we should see somewhere around 3,000 lives saved because of those impacts," Brady said. "Despite expansive training and AED placement in the past 25 years, our nationwide average is still around 10

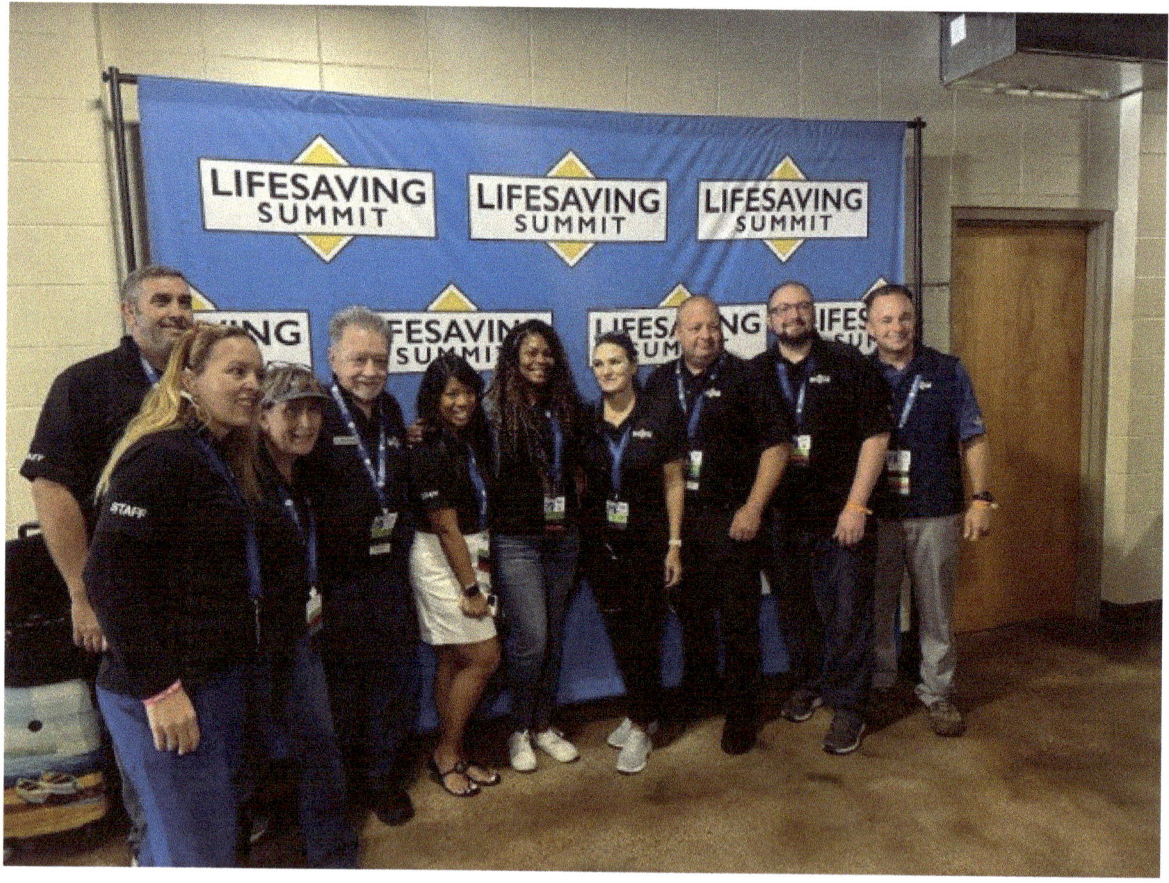

percent for neurologically intact hospital discharge from sudden cardiac arrest—10 percent is not acceptable."

> We have a clear, 10-year target to deliver 1 million lifesaving impacts. For us, that means a student trained, an AED placed, an AED put on program management, or a bleeding control kit installed.
> —Brady McLaughlin, CEO and Founder of GoRescue

When Brady referred to a 10 percent survival rate, he was specifically talking about patients who had out-of-hospital cardiac arrest and survived all the way to hospital discharge with good neurological function. This is considered the gold standard outcome, meaning the person survives and retains meaningful brain function. It's important to note that this figure is an average, and outcomes can vary widely depending on factors such as how quickly CPR is started, whether an AED is used, and where the arrest occurs.

Brady highlighted a critical gap between effort and outcomes in cardiac arrest response. Despite decades of widespread CPR training and increased AED placement, only about 10 percent of patients survive sudden cardiac arrest with good neurological function. His point was not that these efforts are ineffective, but that they are often misaligned—training and equipment are not consistently reaching the environments where cardiac arrests most commonly occur, particularly in the home. As a result, the system as a whole is underperforming, and improving survival will require more strategic placement, better integration, and a shift in how preparedness is delivered.

Within Stop Heart Attack was Bleedingcontrolkits.com, an entity based on the Stop the Bleed initiative, which constructs and distributes their own bleeding control kits nationwide. Bleeding control kits are designed to rapidly address life-threatening hemorrhage and typically include a tourniquet, gauze for wound packing (often hemostatic), and a pressure bandage to maintain bleeding control. Supporting items such as gloves, trauma shears, and a marker are included to assist with safe and effective care, along with basic instructions for use. These kits are intentionally simple and accessible, allowing bystanders to intervene quickly in emergencies where uncontrolled bleeding could otherwise lead to death within minutes.

> Despite expansive training and AED placement in the past 25 years, our nationwide average is still around 10 percent for neurologically intact hospital discharge from sudden cardiac arrest—10 percent is not acceptable.
> —Brady McLaughlin, CEO and Founder of GoRescue

Brady and the entire GoRescue team are passionate and intentional about what they do. The team abides by four core values: honor to God, excellence in service, living in balance, and stewardship through accountability. GoRescue intentionally focuses only on lifesaving solutions that directs the team in culture and business.

Brady explained that the purpose of any business is to solve people's problems. In 2015, he went to an HSI conference where instructors were passionate about CPR and wanted to learn, collaborate, and grow. (I imagine he probably felt much like I did at my first LSS.) HSI is a national training organization that provides CPR, AED, first aid, and safety education programs.

It's one of the main alternatives to the American Heart Association and American Red Cross in the CPR training space.

When that conference ceased to convene, Brady recognized a void and filled it by starting the LSS in 2019, with the clear vision to propel the CPR and AED industry forward by curating a consolidated, powerful experience for CPR instructors, small business leaders, aspiring instructors, and sudden cardiac arrest survivors. This allows for meaningful educational sessions for all business stages, team building, and growth for the CPR community.

Scan to learn more about the Lifesaving Summit.

It was important to GoRescue that the LSS give instructors and businesses a place to learn and excel without competition. They emphasize collaboration over competition, with the attitude that partners can work together and win together.

Each year, LSS is a little different with varying attendees, activities, and topics. In 2025, it was on a cruise to the Bahamas for the first and possibly only time, but it was AMAZING!

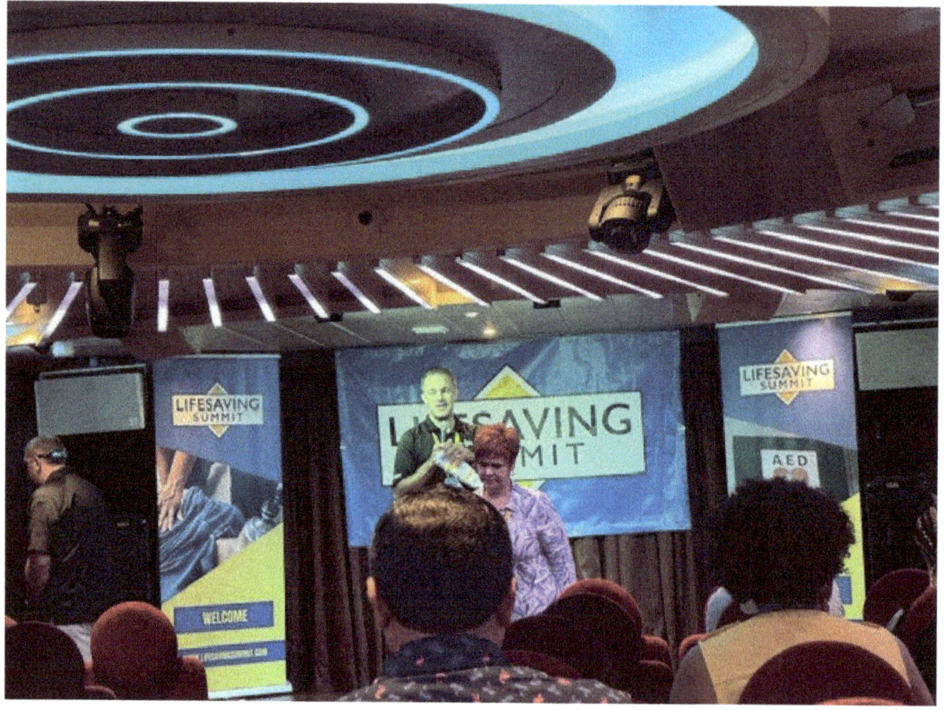

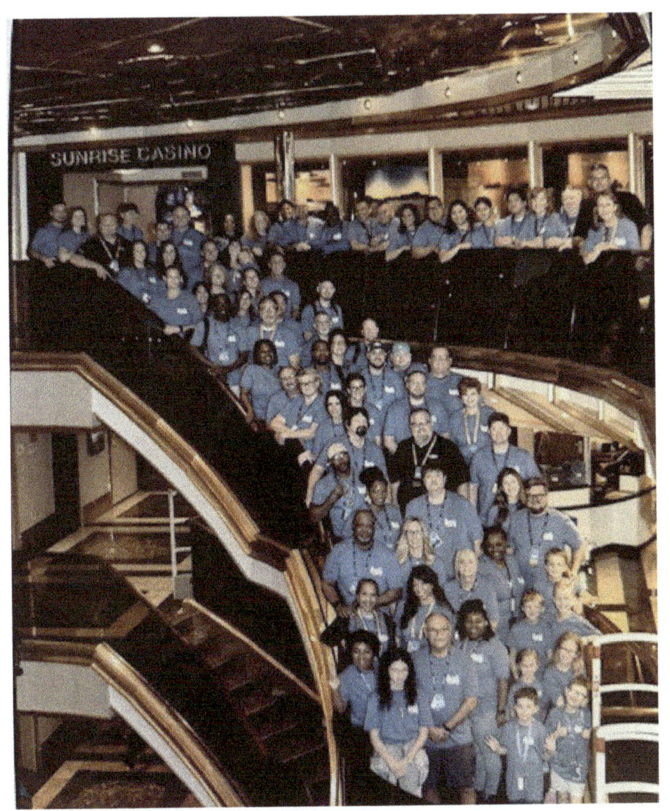
SUNRISE CASINO

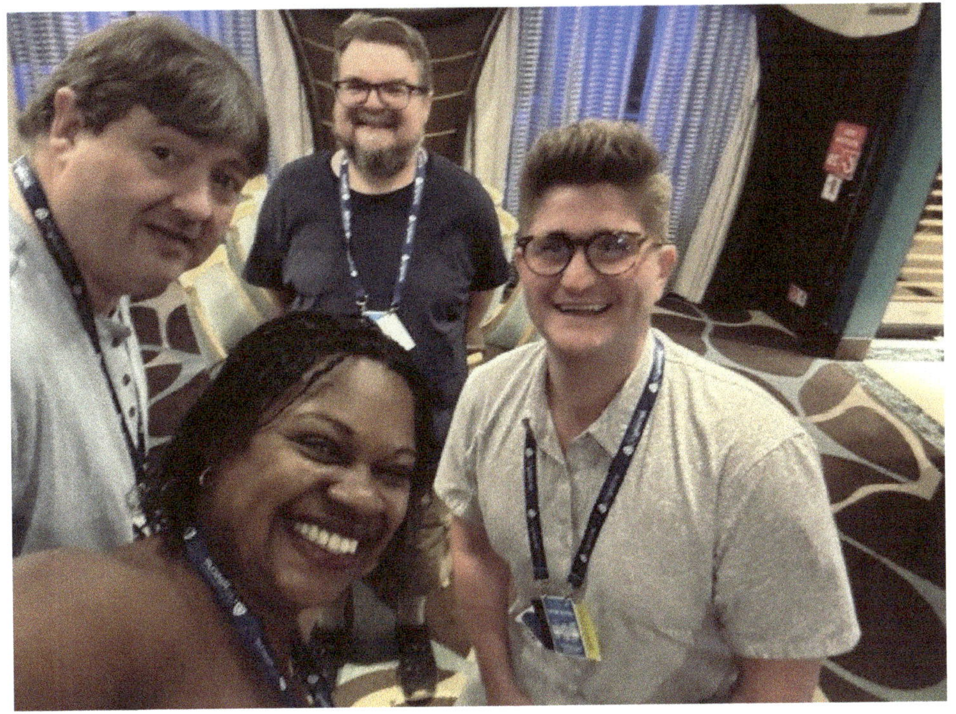

By growing the CPR community, we will all do better at getting the word out about sudden cardiac arrest and related statistics. We inspire one another, and we are there for one another through actual life. People don't always understand entrepreneurs and what we have to do. Sometimes, they don't understand business, and sometimes we don't understand business either. The point is, meeting other entrepreneurs with experience, ideas, and solutions—or just listening ears—can make all the difference in the world. If you make yourself available and do the work, the benefits of the LSS community are tremendous for your business and the CPR and AED industry.

GoRescue is committed to the future expansion of CPR. In 2018, they identified the need for easy-to-use AED program management software, and they created AED 365. AED 365 is evolving consistently to meet industry needs and updates.

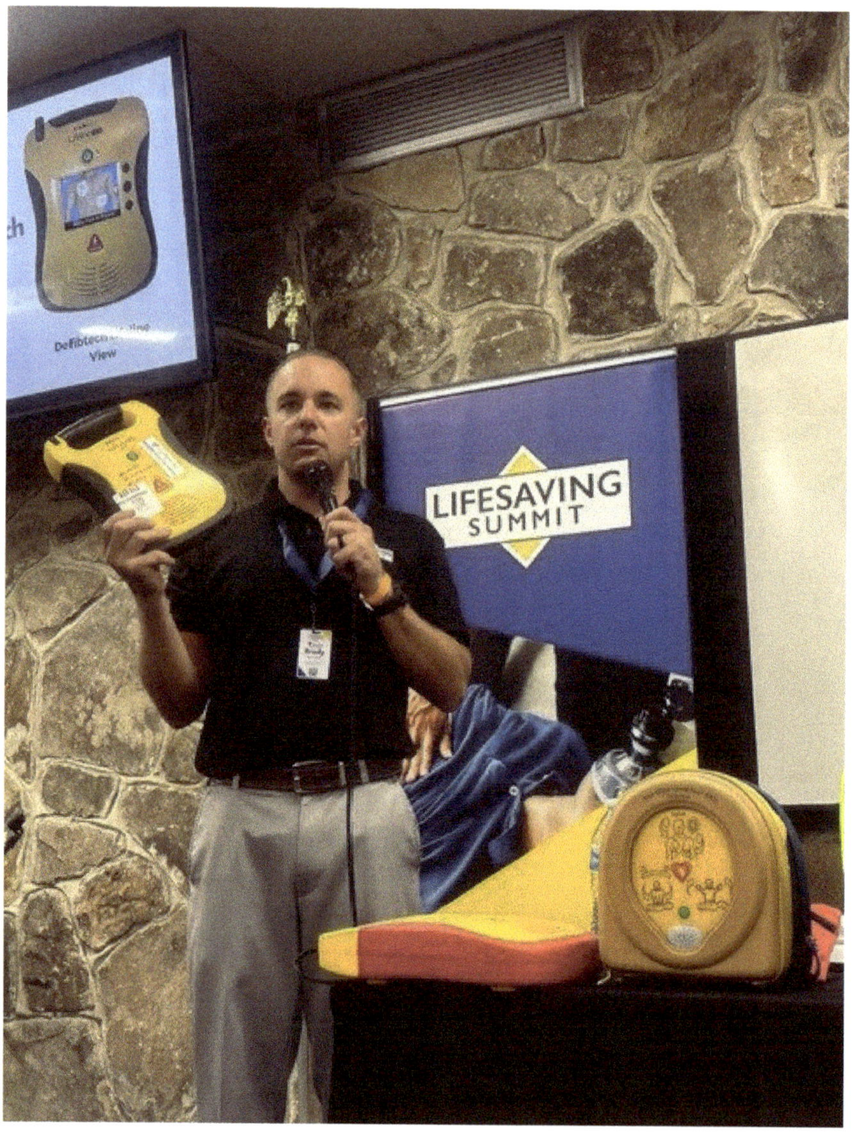

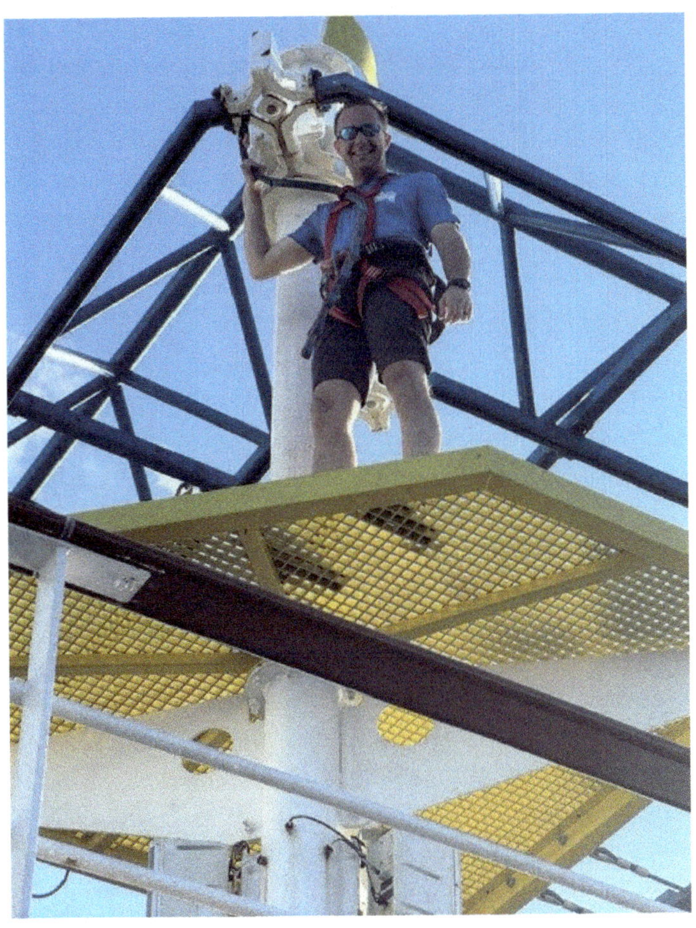

Brady said that after the COVID-19 pandemic, in 2021, about one-third of EMS providers left the industry. He also knew that there was no consolidated, effective training for EMTs—so GoRescue created one, an academy style fast-track program. The program is three weeks long, and students attend class six (long) days a week. During the program, participants develop baseline EMT skills and learn how to work as a team. The curriculum also includes life lessons on personal finance, attention to detail, punctuality, discipline, and time management. The goal is to train a successful EMT and to build a successful community member. I am not sure if either of the colleges I attended cared, LOL.

GoRescue empowers people to help others experiencing sudden cardiac arrest. To date, they have placed more than 35,000 AEDs and trained over 330,000 people. Honestly, when I first started going to the LSS, I had not really thought about even keeping track. I just took pride in providing a high-quality class. They explain that it's as simple as the three Es: If you make something easy, engaging, and effective, you can curate an experience that lasts a lifetime. They help instructors like me grow and engage with others, knowing that together we can increase the survival rate of sudden cardiac arrest outside of the hospital through our separate and joint efforts.

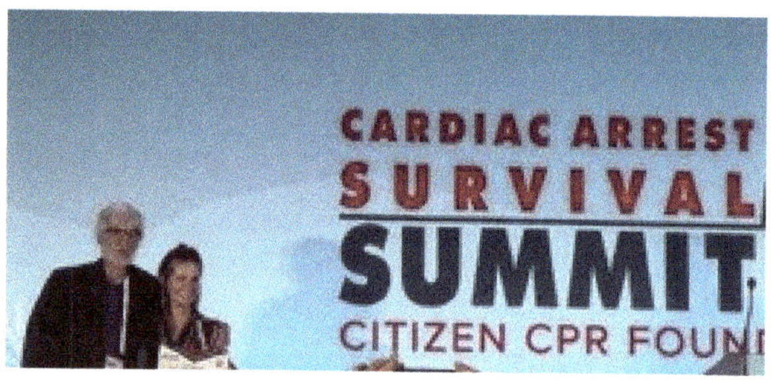

Thanks to my LSS attendance, I have learned about several major events that contribute to advancing the CPR and AED industry forward. Those include the National CPR and AED awareness March and Rally in Washington, D.C; the Cardiac Arrest Survival Summit, hosted biannually by Citizen's CPR; and the Heart to Heart conference organized by Parent Heart Watch.

Another way GoRescue contributes to our CPR community is by sponsoring the ZOLL Summit. Their goal is to assist distribution partners with growth and achievement and help them learn more about ZOLL products and practical strategies to enhance business. Brady stated that futuristically, we have to change the way we deliver AEDs, place AEDs, and deliver CPR.

Brady explained that anyone can be trained on CPR, but rescue-ready AEDs are not in the locations where they are needed most—in homes. The term "rescue-ready" denotes a higher level of readiness. The machines might be the same, but an AED can be placed and not ready to rescue. The pads can be expired, the battery can be expired or near depletion, or the AED itself could be compromised from things like heat and cold exposure. Rescue-ready implies that the AED has been maintained and is actually ready to rescue. Three out of four sudden cardiac arrests happen pre-hospital and most happen in homes. GoRescue has the solution.

"We created a plan to put an AED in a home for as little as a dollar a day, and put AEDs with training in the home for as little as three dollars a day with pediatric functionality," Brady said. Adults and children require different levels of voltage for AED shocks. A model that can save children and adults is ideal for residential use. "We need to get AEDs into homes," Brady continued. "People have to start innovating their businesses to hit that home market. It could be a mix of new business models or lobbying for tax credits, but we have to do something. That will make a difference."

> We need to get AEDs into homes.
> —Brady McLaughlin, CEO and Founder of GoRescue

Chapter 10: The Rhythm of the Movement

Teaching CPR and empowering people with the ability and confidence to perform it—and maybe even save a life—is a privilege. But I would be remiss if I didn't discuss the very real effects that doing CPR can have on people.

We're not just teaching a skill. We're giving people permission to step in when it matters most.
—Cia McClinton, founder of People's Choice CPR

Echoes of the past ring in my head as I think about the first podcast interview I conducted, with Bob Kaplan, who mentioned how CPR Prompt was designed to be an in-home system to guide people through CPR.

GoRescue founder Brady McLaughlin said that's what he believes is needed to seriously decrease sudden cardiac arrest death. I think this entire journey of a story has exemplified that we are all in this world together and should work together for the good of us all learning and benefiting from learning CPR. It could be any of us, any of our loved ones, and someone, anyone can react. It's that simple.

"We're not just teaching a skill. We're giving people permission to step in when it matters most," said Cia McClinton, founder of People's Choice CPR.

This seems so natural for people who want to help, and maybe the reason other people don't act as quickly is the emotional and mental resonance associated with the task. Performing CPR can definitely have lasting effects. Even as a healthcare provider, I have wondered, *Have I performed well enough?*

Another challenge is that many people who perform CPR never hear of the patient's outcome. If you weren't directly caring for that patient, or if they were transferred out of your care, their outcome may forever be unknown. That's as it should be as far as HIPAA goes.

If someone wasn't there to do CPR, the patient probably would have died. You don't think about that until later. Talking about it right now kind of brings it back. It stays with you.
—Stewart Garnett, rescuer and survivor

"If someone wasn't there to do CPR, the patient probably would have died. You don't think about that until later. Talking about it right now kind of brings it back. It stays with you," said Stewart Garnett, who has both saved a person with CPR and survived two sudden cardiac arrests. (Scan the QR code in Chapter 11 to learn more about Stewart Garnett's story.)

Most people would understand that *having* cardiac arrest and receiving CPR would cause mental health effects. But the psychological impact is not limited to survivors. People who *perform* CPR also might experience significant emotional responses.

> I knew mentally I could not watch my son doing CPR on my husband, so I knew that I had to do it.
> —Corrie Williams, rescuer

Research indicates that 25 to 35 percent of lay rescuers report some form of psychological distress following a resuscitation attempt. Among healthcare providers, 10 to 20 percent experience symptoms consistent with PTSD after repeated exposure to resuscitation events.

Many rescuers report acute stress reactions, intrusive memories, and self-doubt about the quality of care they provided. Sensory experiences, such as the physical effort of compressions, sounds during CPR, or visual details of the event, can become chronic memory triggers.

When CPR is performed on a loved one, the psychological impact is often intensified.

"My best friend saw CPR being performed on me. He's still traumatized by it," said Robyn Shore, who experienced a sudden cardiac arrest during her first aid class and was saved by the instructor. Yes, the class was cancelled. (Learn more about Robyn's story in Chapter 11.)

If the rescuer is also a loved one, the rescuer must balance two roles simultaneously: emotional attachment and clinical responsibility.

"I knew mentally I could not watch my son doing CPR on my husband, so I knew that I had to do it," said Corrie Williams.

This dual role can increase stress, contribute to longer-term emotional processing, and in some cases, lead to symptoms consistent with trauma-related disorders.

"The sounds from that day will always be in my head. When I hear those sounds, it's disturbing," Corrie said. (Learn more about Corrie's story in Chapter 11.)

Doing CPR on a loved one can have far-reaching consequences.

"I trauma-coded my dad. It was an unsuccessful resuscitation. Afterward, I was at a crossroads. I thought about either completely giving up my career in EMS or taking it to the next level, said James Fields. (Learn more about James's story in Chapter 11.)

Doing CPR to do what we can do, I realized that we needed a resource, which evolved into my podcast, the Wellness Pulse. It's a kinda a reach, but groove with me for a minute. I had learned and met so many wonderful people at the Lifesaving Summit, and in the early sping of 2025, I thought that it would be cool to pay homage to CPR during National CPR Week. I figured my guests and I could discuss CPR in depth, where we have been, where we are, and where we are going. I thought that if people knew the history and stories of CPR, they would be more inclined to take a CPR class. People love drama and a good story!

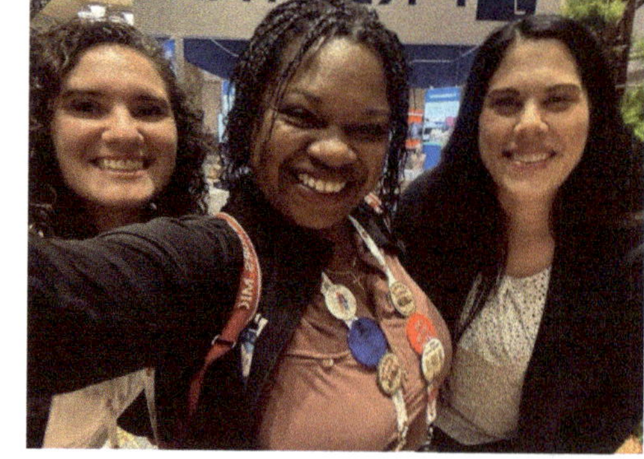

As I began conducting my podcast interviews, the wealth of information was too good to edit into small bites, so I thought that the interviews in their entirety should stand on their own. I was encouraged by my dear friend Lindsay Benz to continue the podcast past National CPR Week. Then I had another epiphany: I needed to also interview people who had been personally affected by sudden cardiac arrest. (I share some of those stories in Chapter 11.) Admittedly, there might be some other subject matter featured on my podcast to support *total* wellness. After all, it is called the Wellness Pulse!

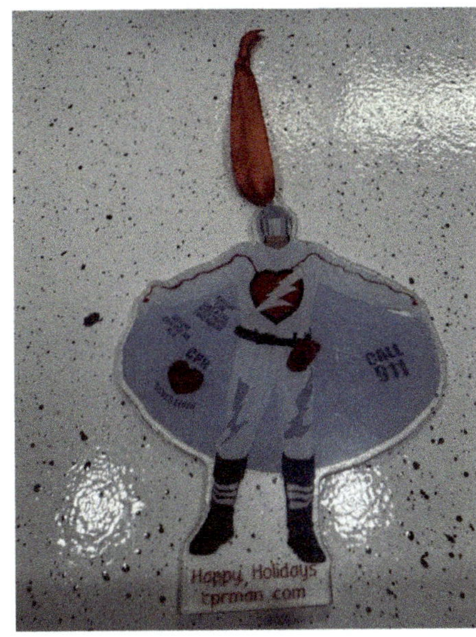

Through taping my podcast and writing this book, I learned about other events that help advocate for and unite CPR crusaders. One of those events is the National CPR and AED Awareness March & Rally in Washington, D.C., organized by Ed Kosiec. Ed is a dear CPR crusader and inspiration, and he is also a superhero of sorts—CPR Man! His work focuses on expanding CPR training, especially among students, and raising awareness of sudden cardiac arrest.

The National CPR and AED Awareness March & Rally is held annually in alignment with National CPR and AED Awareness Week. This multi-day event brings together survivors, advocates, organizations, and the public for CPR demonstrations, advocacy efforts, heart screenings, and large-scale community training. Through both grassroots education and national visibility, Ed's work emphasizes that through bystander readiness anyone can save a life.

On March 12, 2019, what began as a normal day for Ed, with marathon training, yoga, and lunch with his wife in Boynton Beach, Florida, changed when he collapsed from sudden cardiac arrest inside a restaurant. A high school student trained in CPR stepped forward and saved Ed's life.

The Cardiac Arrest Survival Summit (CASS) is another major event, held biannually in collaboration with the Sudden Cardiac Arrest Foundation and the Cardiac Arrest Survivor Alliance. This summit brings together survivors, caregivers, medical professionals, and advocates to explore life after sudden cardiac arrest. The summit provides a space for education, storytelling, and support, focusing on recovery, mental health, and the survival experience.

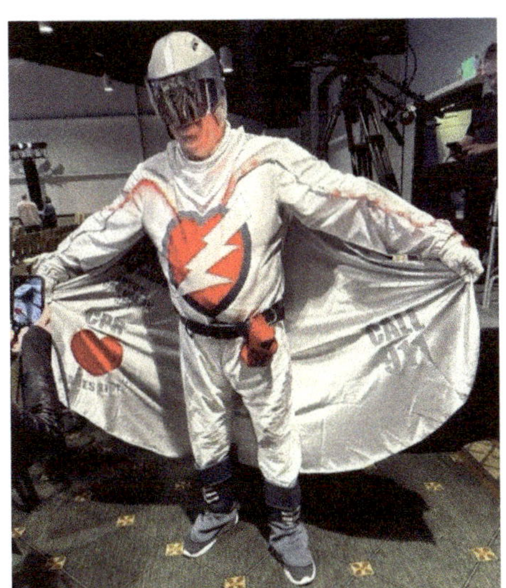

The Sudden Cardiac Arrest Foundation works to improve survival through awareness, education, and community engagement. The Cardiac Arrest Survivor Alliance program supports survivors and families by addressing the emotional and long-term effects of cardiac arrest—emphasizing that survival is only the beginning of recovery.

If you attend the CASS, know that you might not get *all* of that out of the CASS if you come with hyper focus. What do I mean by that? If you come for the academic presentations, they run every day, with

some breakout sessions and time to go to the exhibition floor. Also, scientists, doctors, and advanced practice nurses present the science and share peer-reviewed this and that. In the exhibition hall, you'll find networking opportunities, demonstrations, and the latest and greatest products.

"CASS is a great show for us to connect with instructors and educators, to help them understand what HSI is trying to do to bring CPR training, first aid, and AED training to the market and how we can help grow the industry in total," said Anthony Corwin of Health & Safety Institute (HSI)

Scan to learn more about Huddle for Hearts.

Scan to learn more about the Kyle J Taylor Foundation.

Ah, let's talk about HSI. Remember, this is the company that inspired Brady to start the Lifesaving Summit after the HSI conference ended. HSI embodies the true soul of the entrepreneurial spirit. A contender to the two major American CPR certifying bodies, the American Heart Association and the American Red Cross. "HSI has been around since the 70s, right? We started with Medic First Aid, ASHI, and EMS Safety, and in recent years, we've brought all those programs together to become HSI, which you know today," Anthony said.

ASHI emerged in the mid-1990s as a private-sector response to the growing demand for CPR and first aid training outside traditional institutional settings. Rather than introducing new medical guidelines, it focused on how training could be delivered—providing structured programs that independent instructors and small organizations could use to reach workplaces and community groups. Its development reflects a shift from centralized training models toward more distributed, service-based delivery of lifesaving education. By providing a structured yet flexible program, it allowed independent instructors and small companies to offer CPR and first aid training across a wide range of settings. Its model supported repeatable courses, expanded the customer base beyond healthcare, and gave instructors more control over how training was scheduled and delivered. In that

The Health & Safety Institute has been around from the 70s, right? We started with Medic First Aid, ASHI, and EMS Safety, and in recent years, we've brought all those programs together to become HSI, which you know today.—Anthony Corwin, of HSI sense, ASHI helped move CPR education further into a service-based model, where training could be offered, managed, and grown by individual providers.

EMS Safety Services emerged in the early 2000s as part of a growing shift toward accessible, often online, continuing education for emergency medical professionals. By the time it was acquired by the Health & Safety Institute in 2019, it had become an established provider of training designed to help EMTs and paramedics maintain certification and stay current in their practice.

Scan to learn more about the CASS.

Originally developed as three separate programs across different decades, these training systems were later brought together under HSI through acquisition, forming a unified platform for emergency response education. Together, they formed a more cohesive training ecosystem that supported a wider range of educational needs, from bystander response to professional development. Although entrepreneurship in CPR training had already begun to take shape, this unification made it more practical for some business models to sustain and grow. Instructors and small training companies could operate within a single system, offering multiple types of training without navigating separate organizations. In this way, HSI enhanced the entrepreneurial model by making it easier to deliver, manage, and expand lifesaving education as a service.

Networking, that's the ticket. The inspiration and knowledge I garnered from meeting people at the CASS are priceless. I met people from foundations created in remembrance of their loved ones, such as Huddle for Hearts and the Kyle J Taylor Foundation.

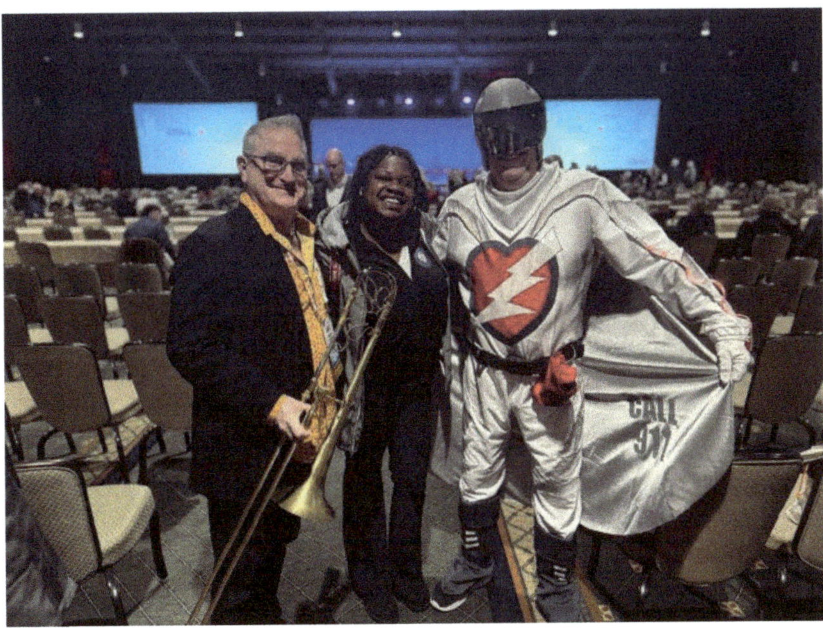

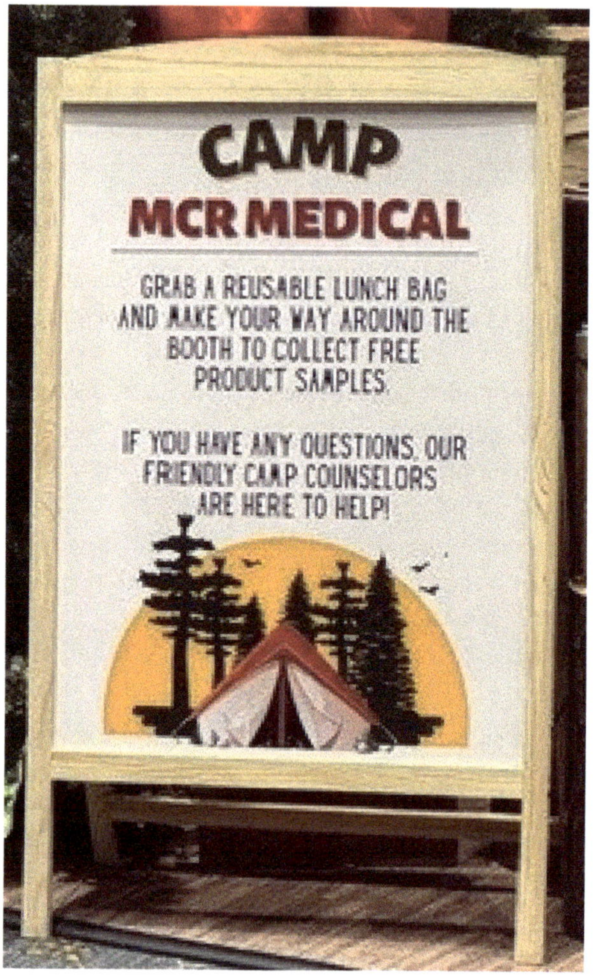

I met new people representing companies I am already acquainted with, such as people from ZOLL. Over at the SafeLife Booth, I saw both new and old faces! I was able to catch up with some of my colleagues and mentors, such as Cheryl Smith of CPR Choice. Artist Maurice Trosclair, also known as "Miracle Meaux," shared about his sudden cardiac arrest, along with his music CD. Others spoke of an upcoming movie, and several books.

I had just been to the Lifesaving Summit a couple weeks prior, so reconnecting with PRESTAN, MCR Medical, HealthForce, and Dr. Fran at the CASS was inspirational. Discovering what other people are doing is motivating. Seeing people so passionate about CPR and discovering ways we can work together is awesome.

MCR Medical did an entire Camp MCR theme! No, the third tract is where survivors mingle, doing dinners and sessions more focused on mental and emotional health. Honestly, I am not sure if they are open to everyone, but I was able to go in as esteemed press. I really bonded with a lot of the attendees, and I was greatly inspired by the advocacy and comrade vibe.

In the CPR community, these events really bring home the point, the *why* we do what we do. Alas, the battle isn't over after we do CPR.

Chapter 11: Between Life and Breath

Sometimes CPR can save lives. Other times, it can't. Still other times, the life might continue, but not in the same rhythm it once knew.

Mental health outcomes following sudden cardiac arrest and resuscitation are well documented. Increasingly, they are recognized as a critical part of recovery. The psychological impact often continues long after the physical event has resolved.

Studies show that 30 to 50 percent of cardiac arrest survivors experience anxiety, depression, or post-traumatic stress. A subset, 15 to 30 percent of them, develop clinically significant post-traumatic stress disorder (PTSD). These symptoms include fear of recurrence, hyper-awareness of bodily sensations such as heart rate, panic episodes, and avoidance of activities that increase physical exertion.

Commonly, survivors experience cognitive changes, including difficulties with memory, attention, and processing. These changes are often associated with temporary reductions in oxygen to the brain during cardiac arrest. Post-intensive care syndrome (PICS) changes include physical, cognitive, and psychological symptoms that can persist for months or even longer.

A key feature of post-cardiac arrest recovery is that psychological symptoms often don't appear until after the patient's discharge, once the immediate crisis has passed. Many people report that they did not initially fully process the severity of the event. Their emotional responses, such as fear, anxiety, or intrusive thoughts, occurred later.

For some survivors, the impact isn't just *what* happened. It's what might happen *next*. The event might be over, but the questions about the future are just beginning.

Sometimes, survivors long to give back to the people who helped them. They are usually deeply grateful to the people and systems that saved their lives.

However, this appreciation does not eliminate the presence of distress. Both can coexist. Overall, current evidence supports the understanding that survival from cardiac arrest is not solely a physical outcome. Psychological recovery is a deeply personal and ongoing, unique process, affecting both survivors and rescuers, and should be recognized as an essential component of post-event care.

Despite these challenges, some people also report post-traumatic growth, including feelings of increased purpose, advocacy, and engagement in education or support efforts.

The CPR stories that follow are not trainings in manuals. They are not captured in survival rates or statistics. These stories illuminate what CPR looks like after the hands leave the chest. They are the part we don't see when we teach it, but they are the reason we teach it at all.

Renee Holmes

I met Renee Holmes, a healthcare IT professional and community leader, at the Blox, an entrepreneurial boot camp. Renee took a sincere interest in my business and CPR, and she took part in the CPR class I taught there.

PRESTAN made sure that I had all the equipment I needed to deliver a high-quality training class while traveling. I used the PRESTAN Ultralites for the first time, and they truly are ultra-light. You get the lights and the click in the chest, minus the weight.

Scan to learn more about Renee's story.

Renee explained that CPR is one of those skills you might never need to use, but at any moment, it can be the difference between life and death.

"I feel the more you know, the faster you can react," Renee said. "The skill level that you have attained in knowing the CPR, knowing exactly what to do and how to do it, and not being hesitant to jump in there and do it are all really, really a big deal."

That reality became deeply personal for Renee when she lost a close friend, who she described as like a brother, to sudden cardiac arrest. There were no warning signs, and afterward those closest to him wished they could have done more. That experience shaped Renee's perspective. "I believe CPR is not just a skill," Renee said. "It's a responsibility."

> I believe CPR is not just a skill. It's a responsibility.
> —Renee Holmes

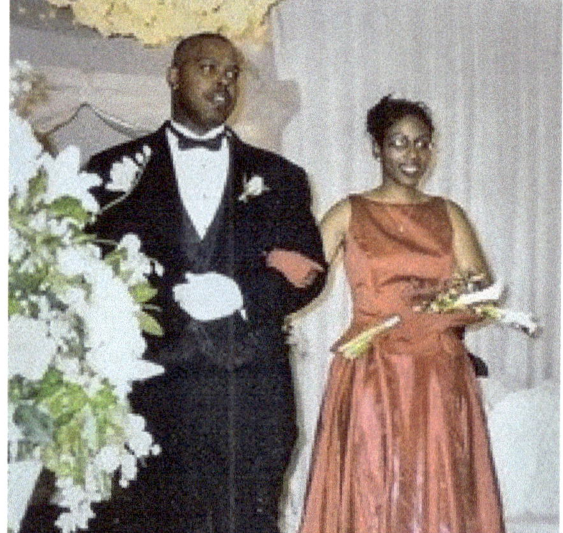

Renee Holmes and the loved one she lost to sudden cardiac arrest

Miranda Burnette

Scan to learn more about Miranda's story.

"CPR is very close to my heart because I want to remember why I started to learn it," Miranda Burnette said.

On September 12, 2008, Miranda Burnette lost her mother-in-law to sudden cardiac arrest. The fire department that responded to Miranda's mother-in-law had a great response time, but the distance from their station to her home was 16 minutes. No one in the home knew how to do CPR, so Miranda's mother-in-law went 16 minutes without any compressions or ventilations to her emergency.

> CPR is very close to my heart because I want to remember why I started to learn it.
> —Miranda Burnette

"I learned CPR to ensure that no one is in that same situation, that their loved one arrives alive at the hospital, is discharged from the hospital, and that they get to spend more time with their family," Miranda said.

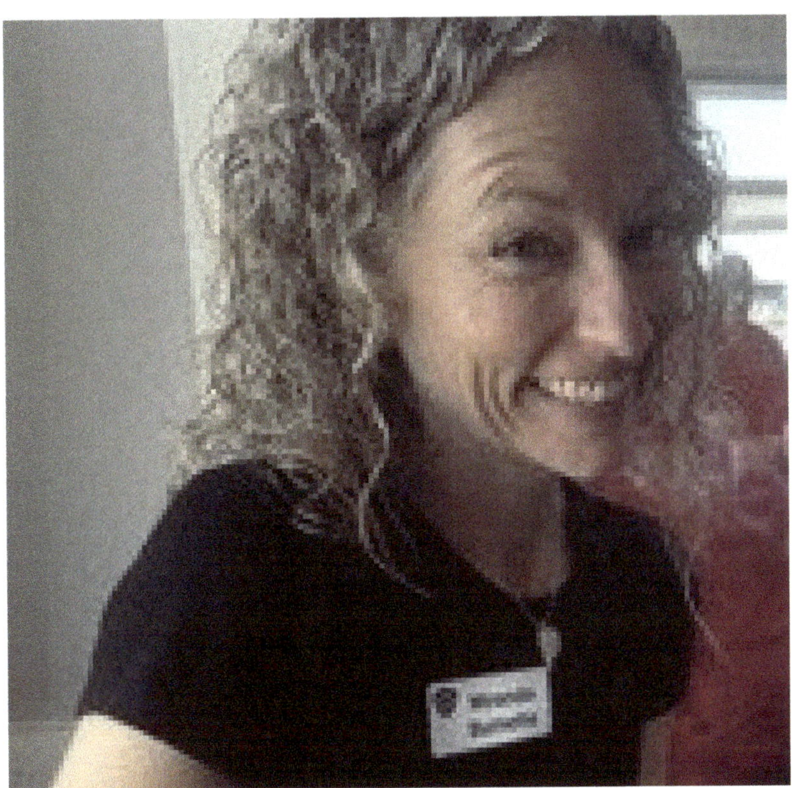

Miranda Burnette

James Fields

Scan to learn more about James's story

"I started in EMS at 13 years old," James Fields said. "It gave me something to do and kept me out of trouble.

James quickly discovered he had a passion for helping people. He's been doing that his entire life. But in 1998, he trauma-coded his own father. It was an unsuccessful resuscitation.

James was at a crossroads. "I thought I could either completely give up EMS, or I could take it to the next level," he said. "I wanted more skills to prevent somebody else from having the same outcome as I had."

Now James treats every patient like they are his own family. "I've done CPR on around 2,000 people, and I've had around 175 successful saves. My last year alone, I had 16 saves," he said.

I've done CPR on around 2,000 people, and I've had around 175 successful saves. My last year alone, I had 16 saves.
—James Fields, rescuer

Today, James teaches the same skills that he uses. "I make sure people are confident," he said.

The loss of his father is at the core of his work—a deeply personal experience that reshaped his perspective, pushed him to pursue greater skill and deeper knowledge, and motivated in him the commitment to ensure other people have a better chance at survival.

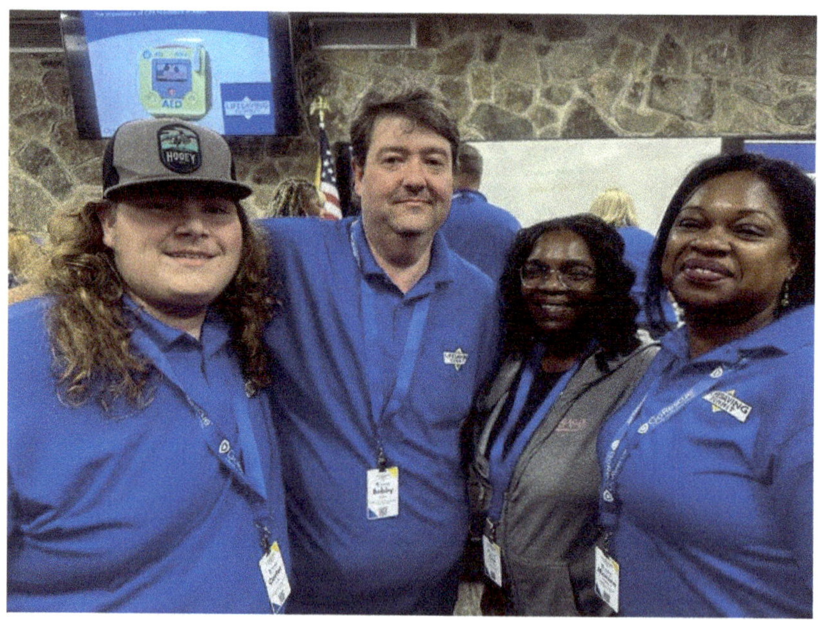

James Fields; his son, Carter; my mother, and me at the Lifesaving Summit 23

Nancy Cordova Wells

A lifelong runner, Nancy Cordova Wells got regular medical checkups and managed known conditions, including high blood pressure. However, subtle warning signs, like abnormal heart rate spikes, were present long before her cardiac event. In the months leading up to her arrest, Nancy experienced a series of medical challenges, including an anaphylactic reaction and the emotional toll of losing her mother just days before her daughter's wedding.

Scan to learn more about Nancy's story.

Despite those stressors, Nancy continued training and preparing for a half-marathon.

On race day, something felt off. What began as mild discomfort progressed into distress, but Nancy pushed forward, attributing it to environmental conditions.

Nancy doesn't remember a step beyond mile four and a half. She woke up in a hospital, learning she had suffered a cardiac arrest caused by a blockage in her left anterior descending artery, which is often called the "widow maker." Immediate CPR from a bystander nurse and defibrillation efforts by emergency responders restored her heartbeat.

"A piece of plaque got lodged in my artery," Nancy said. "They told me that I didn't have a pulse for 10 minutes." During that time, Nancy recalls a vivid experience—seeing a bright light and her mother telling her it was not yet her time.

Nancy's recovery was rapid, going from the intensive care unit to walking within days. She defied typical expectations. Still, the emotional aftermath included confusion, anger, and the question of "why me," especially given her active lifestyle.

"I was kind of a little angry," Nancy said.

They told me that I didn't have a pulse for 10 minutes.—Nancy Cordova Wells (During that time, Nancy recalls a vivid experience—seeing a bright light and her mother telling her it was not yet her time.)

But as time passed, Nancy reframed her experience as a turning point. She made lifestyle changes, left a toxic work environment, and focused on her well-being. She also became an advocate, sharing her story to highlight the importance of CPR, especially for women, who statistically receive less bystander intervention. Her message is clear: Survival often depends on someone being willing to act. In Nancy's case, that willingness made the difference between life and death.

"I wouldn't be sitting here today if people hadn't jumped in," Nancy said

Corrie and Jason Williams

Scan to learn more Corrie and Jason story.

When Corrie Williams was a teenager, she was trained in CPR, never knowing when, or if, she would need to use it. One day at the hardware store where Corrie worked, she was alerted that a gentleman had collapsed in the parking lot and was unresponsive. She gave rescue breaths, and two coworkers joined her. The team continued until medics arrived.

"He pulled through," Corrie said. "They shocked him and brought him back."

Decades later, Corrie's training again became critical when her husband, Jason, suddenly collapsed at home.

> I was 48 with no medical history, and I just dropped.
> —Jason Williams

"I was 48 with no medical history, and I just dropped," Jason said. "The day before, I had a strange feeling in my chest—like a thumb pressing—but it went away with Tums. I woke up early in the morning with that same feeling, so I went downstairs and took Tums again."

Jason doesn't remember it, but somehow he climbed back up the stairs, then collapsed just feet away from Corrie, who woke to the sound of him falling. At first, she called out to him, expecting a normal response, but instead she heard something that told her something was terribly wrong.

When Corrie reached Jason, he was gasping and barely breathing. She called 911, put the phone on speaker, and went straight into action.

Their son, who had recently been CPR certified through lifeguard training, came upstairs and asked what he could do. Corrie was grateful he could back her up, but she wanted to be the one to do compressions. "I could not watch my son doing CPR on my husband," Corrie said. "I knew I could not handle that."

Together, Corrie and her son moved Jason into the doorway so she could position herself correctly. The 911 operator instructed her to do compressions only.

What followed was relentless. Corrie remembers the physical force it took and the sounds, sweat, panic, profanity, adrenaline, and determination that drove her. She kept going hard and fast, trying to sustain James until help arrived.

As Corrie did CPR, she repeated to her husband, "You can't do this to me. You're not gonna die on me."

Corrie performed CPR for just under 15 minutes before paramedics arrived. Even after the medics arrived, Corrie stayed locked into the reality of the moment. She watched them shock her husband. She asked where they were taking him. She called family. On the drive to the hospital, she was convinced he was gone. She told their son over and over, "He's dead."

At the hospital, Corrie saw Jason alive, and the surrealness of that reversal never really left either of them. When Jason first became aware enough to understand what had happened, he was told plainly, "You died. Your wife saved your life with CPR."

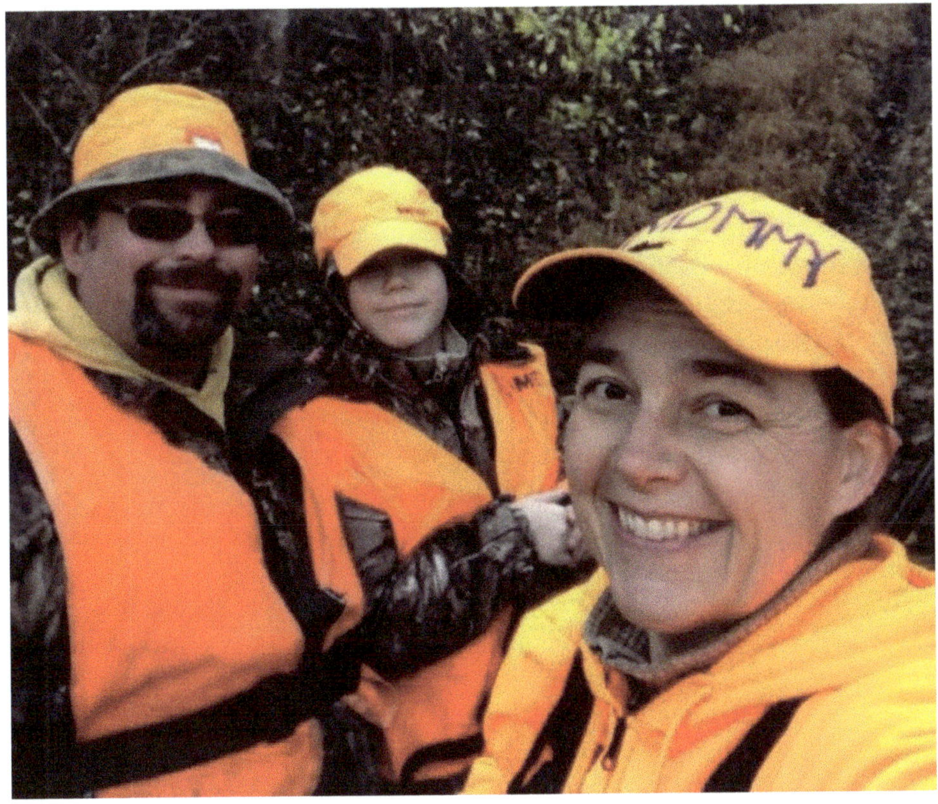

Corrie Williams, Jason Williams, and their son

Later, Jason received an implantable cardioverter defibrillator. He learned that his cardiac event had been caused by ventricular fibrillation (VF) rather than blocked arteries.

Jason's recovery brought a whole new set of realities—physical pain, interrupted sleep, fear, uncertainty, and the emotional aftershock that followed the entire family home. "The mental aspect afterward is something people don't even discuss," Jason said.

He does not believe he carries post-traumatic stress disorder (PTSD), but he is very clear that Corrie does. "She has substantial PTSD," he said.

Neither Corrie nor Jason hesitates to share the message they want others to hear. "If you don't react, you're not going to do anything. If you react in some way, you're at least making an attempt."

To this day, Corrie watches people closely in public, pays attention to distress, and believes hesitation is the greatest danger. Her conviction is as clear now as it was in the moment she saved Jason's life.

From the other side of survival, Jason adds the perspective only someone who has survived sudden cardiac arrest can give. "Don't assume cardiac arrest can only happen to someone else. Don't live in fear, but do be ready."

Corrie and Jason now want to become CPR instructors themselves to help other people learn the skill that saved Jason's life.

"The worst CPR is no CPR," Corrie said.

Stewart Garnett

Scan to learn more about Stewart's story.

"I've had two cardiac arrests," Stewart Garnett said. "The first one was at the YMCA playing basketball. Thank God there was a firefighter and an AED nearby."

Stewart's second sudden cardiac arrest occurred at his home. Blessedly, he lived across the street from the fire department and received advanced care very quickly.

After Stewart's recovery, he returned to his work as a bartender, which he has been doing for more than 30 years. He's even saved several people from choking.

Stewart is also a lay rescuer. One day, he was walking downtown in Winnipeg, Manitoba, Canada, when a gentleman about 10 feet in front of him collapsed and went into cardiac arrest, right in front of the Woodbine Bar, where Stewart was going to meet his dad.

"The man's girlfriend was freaking out," Stewart said. "I called 911, and I learned CPR in about three minutes. The helpful dispatcher guided me through. Another gentleman held the phone next to my face so I could hear while I was giving CPR. I didn't have to give the man mouth-to-mouth, but I pumped him for about four minutes, then the fire department came and took him away. To actually see the gentleman come back out of it—to have pumped him back to life was emotional stuff. It gave me an eye-opener on what frontline people do every day."

Stewart continued, "The firefighters gave me credit. They said it's called a 'save.' But I just happened to be at the right place at the right time. I still see that man's dad once in a while downtown. He always shakes my hand and gets a little teary-eyed. It's nice to have him appreciate what I did for his son."

Sierra Hoffines and Carl Shirtzinger and Rescuers Earl Ehrhart, Daryl Mobley, Tom Agnew, and Andrew Smock

Scan to learn more about Sierra's story.

There was no sign that everything was about to go haywire," said Sierra Hoffines, another fellow Bloxer and environmental IT entrepreneur. Her CPR story hit me super close to home. If her adoptive uncles had not stepped in, her dad would not be here to cherish moments with her son, Gideon. Sierra's father, Carl, was rescued by his coworkers Andrew Smock, Darrell Mobley, Tom Agnew, and Earl Ehrhart.

Sierra's father, a NASA engineer for more than 25 years, had been active in their family group chat leading up to his sudden cardiac arrest, sharing photos and updates about projects he was working on around the house. From Sierra's perspective, everything appeared to be normal.

Earl explained that the day Carl had his sudden cardiac arrest at work had been ordinary—until someone ran into the morning meeting and exclaimed that Carl was unresponsive in the bathroom. When Earl ran into the bathroom, he found Carl in a stall, non-responsive, purple, and without a pulse. Earl kicked in the stall door, then he moved Carl to the floor, sent someone for the AED, and immediately began compressions.

As more coworkers arrived in the bathroom, they took turns doing compressions as they became tired. After the AED arrived, they used it when it advised a shock. Earl said the experience was physical and real and that he could tell they were hurting Carl, likely breaking bones, but they also began to see signs of improvement as Carl's color started coming back and he began making sounds like he was trying to come to. Earl remembered that time felt distorted, that "it felt like 30 seconds" while it was happening, and that once Carl was in the ambulance he felt a "dump of adrenaline."

> There was no sign that everything was about to go haywire.
> —Sierra Hoffines, an environmental IT entrepreneur

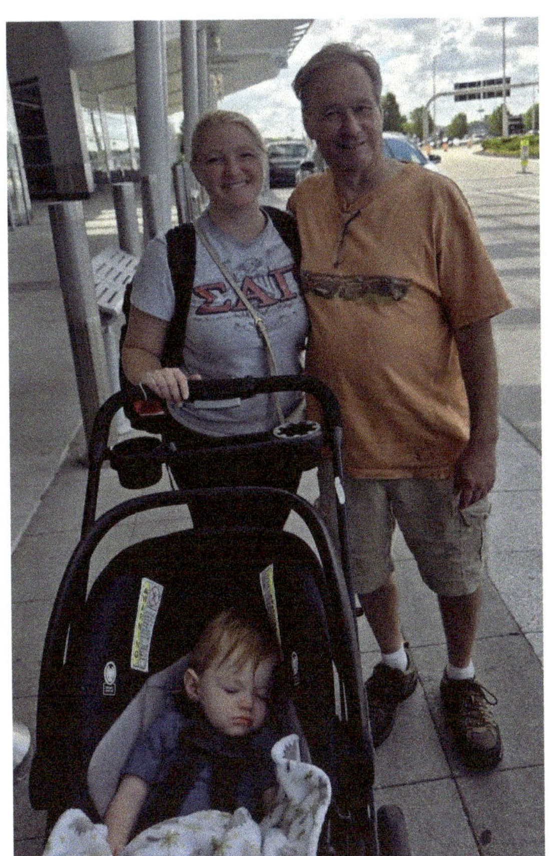

Sierra Hoffines; her father, Carl Shirtzinger; and her son

Another one of their coworkers, Daryl, added that he had spoken to Carl not long before the event, so seeing him on the floor was especially jarring. When Daryl entered the bathroom, Earl already had the AED on Carl, who was "purple as can be." The AED gave them feedback on whether or not they were compressing hard enough. For Daryl, one of the hardest parts was feeling the resistance change in Carl's chest as they continued working, which made him question if he was pressing hard enough even while the AED guided him.

When the third coworker, Tom, took a turn doing compressions, the AED kept telling him to push harder. But Tom felt like he was already giving it everything he had. That made it clear to Tom how different *real* CPR is from training. In class, you practice on manikins, but now Tom was working on someone he knew. He realized "you can't hurt them" by pushing hard because that is what is required to circulate blood.

The account by the fourth coworker, Andrew, adds another layer. He happened to see the maintenance supervisor running with the AED, realized something serious was happening, and followed because of his medical background. When Andrew walked in and saw Carl "bluer than blue can be," he joined the rotation with the other men.

When I spoke with Carl, his daughter, and his four rescuers, Carl heard some of these rescue details for what seemed like the first time. His memory of the event itself is largely absent. A lot of his hospital memories are vague, and much of what he knows is based on what other people told him about what happened.

Carl remembers going to the bathroom before the meeting, then waking up in the hospital days later. As the men described the stall, the door being kicked in, Carl's color, the compressions, the yelling, and Carl's first responses, I could tell that Carl did not recall any of those details.

Carl's daughter, Sierra, learned about the timeline from both the coworkers and the paramedics. She stated that it took approximately eight minutes from the time emergency services were called for them to arrive at the building, and they estimated it was at least twelve minutes before they physically reached her father. During that time, Carl's survival depended entirely on the people around him.

Sierra coordinated communication with family members. She contacted her siblings, their mother, and other relatives, while also trying to gather information from her father's coworkers who were present during the incident. Because Sierra was not immediately local, she also found someone who could be with her father at the hospital until she arrived. She divided her focus between understanding her father's condition, coordinating with medical staff, and maintaining communication with family.

When Carl arrived at the hospital, he was taken to the cath lab. It was determined that he had not experienced a traditional heart attack, but instead a heart block, which is an electrical issue where the upper and lower chambers of the heart are not working together. Carl was sedated for several days and required ventilatory support. He underwent imaging, including scans to assess for potential brain injury.

Considering the length of time Carl was unresponsive, brain damage was a concern. Doctors informed Sierra there was no evidence of brain damage. One physician specifically emphasized the importance of the CPR performed prior to Carl's hospital arrival, noting that it was a key factor in preserving his brain function.

"I remember the doctor calling and saying, 'We have no idea how your dad doesn't have brain damage. It's a miracle. You need to thank whoever performed CPR,'" Sierra said. "I was told that if CPR and the AED had not been used before paramedics arrived, my father would not have survived." This established that Carl's positive outcome was determined *before* EMS arrival. Sierra calls Earl, Daryl, Tom, and Andrew "guardian angels and uncles" now because their quick action is the reason her father is still alive and neurologically intact.

> I remember the doctor calling and saying, "We have no idea how your dad doesn't have brain damage. It's a miracle. You need to thank whoever performed CPR."
> — Sierra Hoffines,
> an environmental IT entrepreneur

After Carl was under sedation for a few days, he regained consciousness unexpectedly. Sierra had arrived for a visit and saw him struggling because his airway support was still in place. Immediately, she alerted the nursing staff.

During Carl's initial period of awareness, he attempted to communicate by writing. When he wrote, "What hap?" Sierra assessed that he could read, write, spell, and understand communication. With an alphabet board, Carl was able to point to letters and form words, which confirmed to Sierra that his cognitive function had been preserved.

When the rescuers were asked about their mental recovery post-CPR, their responses varied. Daryl explained that the hardest part was going home that night and replaying it, wondering if they had done everything right and whether or not there was anything else they could have done. He added, "The key is to get CPR training because once you have CPR training, instinct takes over."

Earl agreed, saying he kept replaying those 10 minutes over and over again in his head. He said the worst part was the unknown, especially before the updates began to come in, noting, "In real life, especially in a prolonged event, multiple trained people are critical because one person alone might not physically be able to keep going long enough."

Andrew said he was praying for Carl that night and continued thinking about it afterward. He was proud of the way they all worked together, noting that when one person tired, another stepped in without hesitation. Also he added, "It is better to know CPR and hopefully never use it than to need it and not know what to do."

Tom said that after the paramedics arrived and took over, he and Daryl were physically stuck in the bathroom and had to stand there watching the professionals continue the code. That gave him the chance to compare what they had done with what the paramedics were doing, which reassured him that they had been doing compressions correctly. He said, "People should learn CPR because emergencies are unexpected, and the basics matter until professionals arrive."

Together, their comments showed that even when a rescue goes well, the responders still carry the mental burden of wondering whether they did enough.

Meanwhile, Carl said his own lingering physical reminder was the eight fractured ribs. But he is "not complaining," which underscores that the painful consequences of effective CPR were secondary to survival.

Robyn Shore

Scan to learn more about Robyn's story.

The day of Robyn's cardiac arrest began as a routine first aid training session with her colleagues. "We went to the course, and I volunteered to get on the floor and do the recovery position. I was overacting, getting up and saying, 'Look at me! I was dead.' Then I felt dizzy, sat down, and thought, *I feel a bit weird.*"

Then—blackness.

Because of Robyn's behavior during the training, her coworkers initially believed she was still acting. Later, she learned that people reported she was making noises, and those around her assumed it was part of her class dramatization, until the instructor recognized that the situation had become serious. The instructor assessed Robyn, immediately identified the problem, stated, "No. She's purple," and began CPR without delay.

The instructor continued CPR and declined offers from other people to take over, believing she was the most capable person in the room to perform it correctly. Robyn attributes her positive outcome, including the absence of major brain injury, to that decision and the quality of CPR provided.

The next memory Robin has is regaining consciousness with emergency responders around her. "I said, 'Oh, I'm so sorry, I need to get up,' because I thought I had just fainted. And one of the EMTs said, 'No ma'am.' I will always remember that," Robyn said. "I'd never been called ma'am before."

> I thanked her and bought her chocolate.
> —Robyn Shore, upon meeting the instructor who performed CPR.

Robyn stated that she lost memory again shortly after that, then woke up in the emergency department, drenched in sweat and experiencing chest discomfort, which she later understood was related to CPR. Initially, she believed she would be discharged after having what she thought was a fainting episode, but further evaluation revealed that she had experienced a cardiac arrest caused by an arrhythmia rather than a heart attack.

Robyn underwent multiple tests and monitoring, with several days spent adjusting medications to stabilize her heart rhythm. Eventually, she had additional procedures, including an angiogram, and she was advised to have an implantable cardioverter defibrillator (ICD) placed. She reflected that she wishes she had undergone an MRI prior to receiving the device because her current device limits that option, and she feels there are still unanswered questions about the extent of any underlying damage.

Following discharge, Robyn transitioned into ongoing follow-up care, including regular ICD checks, cardiology visits, and imaging such as echocardiograms. Over time, her heart has been improving, and her providers are satisfied with her progress.

Later, Robyn met the instructor who performed CPR. "I thanked her and bought her chocolate," she said.

When discussing the importance of bystander CPR, Robyn speaks very directly from her experience, emphasizing that her survival depended entirely on someone recognizing the situation and acting immediately.

"If I hadn't been with somebody that knew what to do, I would not be here anymore."

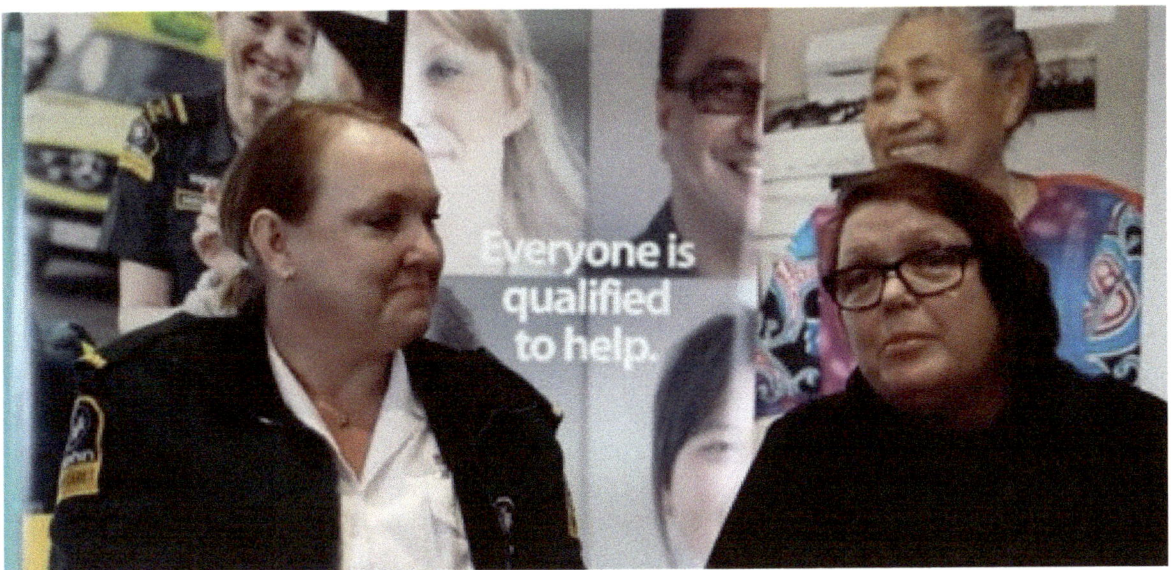

Robyn Shore and her rescuer

Lindsay Sherwood

When I connected with Lindsay Sherwood, she explained that even though she had a known heart condition, her cardiac arrest still occurred in a way that she did not anticipate.

"I'm a 39-year-old female, a single mom of two boys. Years ago, I was diagnosed with an electrical condition of the heart called CVPT. I was on medication for 20 years without any issues. I was living life just great for a long time with regular follow-ups and reassurance from my cardiologist that as long as I remained compliant with treatment, I would be fine."

Scan to learn more about Lindsay's story.

Just two weeks prior to Lindsay's cardiac arrest, she had undergone testing, including a stress test, blood work, and an ECG, all of which were normal, reinforcing that there was no immediate indication that an event was about to occur.

Admittedly, the circumstances surrounding Lindsay's cardiac arrest involved a combination of physical and emotional stressors—enough to give someone even *without* a heart condition a cardiac event. Lindsay was simultaneously moving and dealing with a family crisis in which her brother-in-law had gone missing. After two days of family and friends searching, a search team was called in. Lindsay was with family members when they received the news regarding his situation. Within two minutes of hearing the news, Lindsay collapsed. She has no memory of what occurred after that.

The presence of trained responders at that moment made the difference in Lindsay's survival. Immediately, they began resuscitation efforts. Lindsay received 31 minutes of CPR, during which time she also experienced a stroke. She was transported to the hospital and remained in a coma for three days. Her recovery involved both neurological and physical challenges, including broken ribs and sternum from CPR, but she emphasizes that despite the severity of the event, she regained consciousness and was able to recover to the point of telling her story.

After Lindsay's recovery, she met with the officers involved in her resuscitation. "They were shocked that I pulled through. They said they had a hard time bringing me back. At the time, they didn't think I would survive," Linday said, explaining that one of the officers on scene had a personal AED and had that not been available in that moment, the outcome likely would have been different.

In the hospital, Lindsay learned that her cardiac arrest was not caused by a heart attack, but rather related to the electrical nature of her condition, which is influenced by adrenaline. The extreme stress she was under at the time likely triggered the cardiac event. As part of her treatment, she had an implantable cardioverter defibrillator (ICD) placed, which is expected to manage future risk related to her arrhythmia.

Before the event, Lindsay did not think about needing to know CPR or advocating for other people to be trained. Because she had been stable for many years and had been reassured medically, she did not fully understand the degree of risk.

> I started working with the officers to get more defibrillators placed in rural areas and to increase awareness about them because the only reason I survived was that one officer had his own personal defibrillator. If the officer hadn't had that, it wouldn't have been a good outcome.
> —Lindsay Sherwood

After the event, Lindsay recognized that even with monitoring and normal test results, a sudden cardiac arrest can still occur without warning. She acknowledged that even after people learn CPR, they might not feel confident in their skills. That is how she felt, but today she encourages other people to get CPR training regardless of hesitation, stating that fear or uncertainty should not prevent someone from learning or acting.

Lindsay's experience reinforces that survival is often dependent on what happens before EMS arrives, and both knowledge and equipment play a role in that window of time. Today, Lindsay is actively involved in efforts to increase access to AEDs, particularly in rural areas where emergency response times might be longer.

"I started working with the officers to get more defibrillators placed in rural areas and to increase awareness about them because the only reason I survived was that one officer had his own personal defibrillator. If the officer hadn't had that, it wouldn't have been a good outcome," Lindsay said.

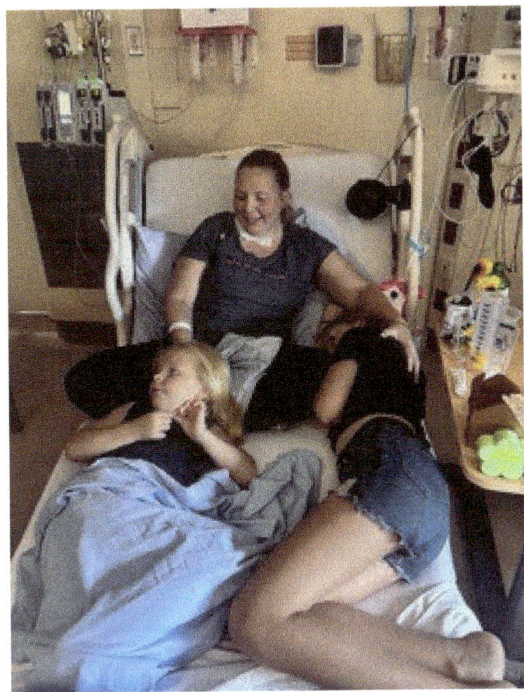

Lindsay Sherwood and her family

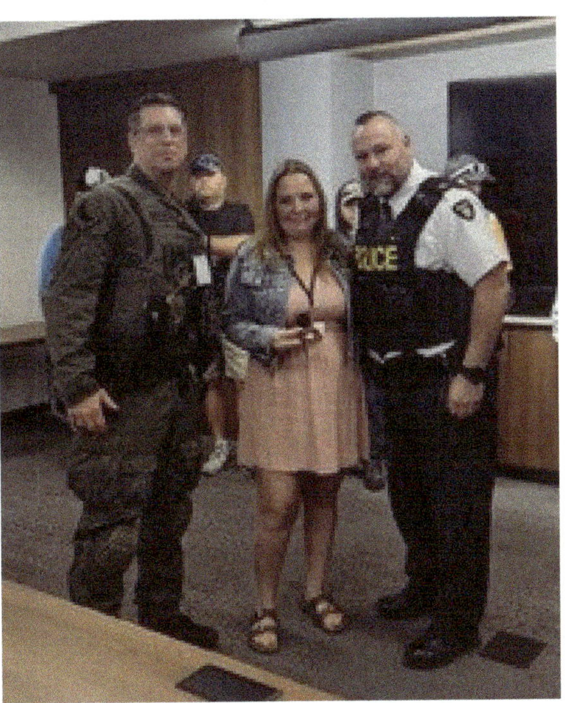

Lindsay Sherwood and her rescuers

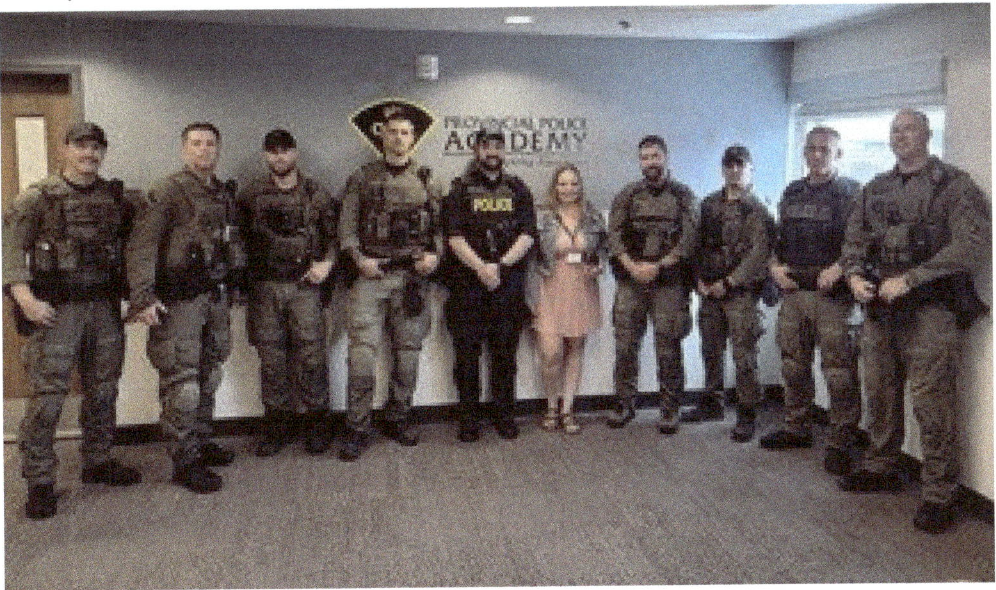

Lindsay Sherwood and her rescuers

Rob Kalmowitz

Scan to learn more about Rob's story.

Up until Rob Kalmowitz's first cardiac event, he had been active, regularly exercising and maintaining what he believed was a relatively healthy lifestyle. Just days before his first cardiac arrest, he and his wife had taken a trip to Atlantic City, New Jersey, to celebrate their engagement anniversary, spending the weekend together without any major concerns.

Even after they returned home, everything followed a typical routine—unpacking, eating dinner, and preparing to relax for the evening. Rob felt mild discomfort in his stomach, which he attributed to something he had eaten. "I came into the bedroom, got a glass of water because my stomach didn't feel right, and sat on the bed. The last thing I remember saying was, 'Connie, I don't feel good.'"

The rest of the event was reconstructed through what Rob's family told him. His wife immediately recognized that something was wrong when he collapsed and was not breathing. She called out to their son, who responded quickly, calling 911 and beginning CPR right away.

> The last thing I remember saying was, "Connie, I don't feel good."
> —Rob Kalmowitz

Their son, who had taken a CPR course years earlier for a college credit, stepped in without hesitation, while his wife and the 911 operator provided guidance. Rob was moved to the floor to allow for proper compressions, and shortly after, police arrived with an AED. Within minutes of receiving CPR and a shock, Rob was resuscitated.

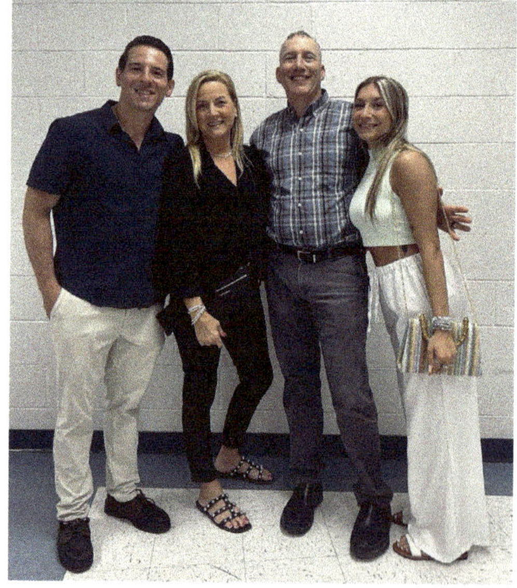

Rob Kalmowitz and family

Rob went into cardiac arrest at 8:08 PM, and after one shock he was back at 8:17.

Rob describes this first event as life-altering but difficult to fully comprehend and process. He did not immediately grasp the severity of what had happened and hoped to return to normal activities quickly.

However, just days after being discharged from the hospital, a second event occurred. During a cardiology visit, Rob's resting heart rate was significantly elevated, prompting concern. Despite attempts to stabilize him with medication, his condition deteriorated, leading to hospitalization. During further testing, including an MRI, he began experiencing extreme symptoms again. He recalls seeing his heart rate on a monitor at 264 beats per minute and thinking, *I'm in trouble.*

Then he lost consciousness for a second time.

Later, Rob learned that a nurse initiated CPR immediately and that he was blessedly again resuscitated within minutes using defibrillation. Following this second cardiac arrest, his understanding of the situation shifted drastically. Unlike the first time, he now fully recognized the seriousness of what had happened, which led to fear and anxiety about his condition and the possibility of recurrence. He explained that surviving two cardiac arrests in such a short period forced him to confront both the physical and psychological impacts of the experience.

Rob described his recovery as having two distinct components: physical and mental. Physically, he was able to rebuild his strength over several months, gradually increasing his activity level from only a few minutes of walking to returning to his baseline.

Mentally, however, the recovery was more complex. Rob experienced panic attacks, fear over his heart rate, and a persistent sense of vulnerability. He avoided leaving his home, viewing it as a place of safety, but he gradually reintroduced himself to normal activities through exposure. He explained that even normal increases in heart rate caused distress because he associated it with the onset of his cardiac events. "If my heart rate hit 100, I thought I was going back to the hospital," he said.

Rob sought professional help and was introduced to concepts such as post-traumatic stress disorder and post-intensive care syndrome, which helped him understand his reactions. Through therapy, journaling, meditation, and other techniques, he began to work through the psychological effects of his experience. As time passed, he developed coping strategies that allowed him to manage his anxiety and regain confidence in his ability to function day to day.

A significant part of Rob's recovery involved connecting with others. He met with the emergency responders who helped save his life, creating a rare opportunity for both survivor and rescuers to come together.

"On my one-year anniversary, my daughter arranged for the EMTs and paramedics to come to my house," Rob said. "We sat together and ate, and I got to thank them. They told me that almost never happens. They don't usually know what happens to the people they save."

Juliana Kalmowitz reflected on how her father's recovery journey was shaped by physical healing and also by the emotional weight that followed the experience. She described moments of fear, anxiety, and vulnerability, noting that even when he appeared physically okay, sometimes he became quieter and more withdrawn as he processed everything mentally and emotionally. Through it all, she saw her role as simply being present—listening without judgment, offering reassurance, and making sure he never felt alone.

"I want people to understand that recovery isn't just physical. It's mental and emotional too. Those parts can be just as hard, if not harder. Supporting a survivor means being patient and present and understanding that healing doesn't happen in a straight line," Juliana said.

That experience led Rob to create a support group focused on mental health for cardiac arrest survivors, Sudden Cardiac Arrest Survivor Mental Health Awareness.

"I needed help not just physically, but mentally. I went to therapy and learned ways to deal with the trauma. That's one of the biggest things that aren't discussed, for survivors and co-survivors. I created my support group to help people dealing with these mental health challenges," Rob said.

I find that to be typical of the medical practice in the United States, where mental health is not always prioritized. I was truly touched to stumble upon survivors in Rob's support group. I value total wellness encompassing mind, body, and spirit, so seeing support groups for people who have gone through sudden cardiac arrest was inspiring. I met great people in Rob's group. Unless a person has had a sudden cardiac arrest or knows someone who has, the challenges associated with it can be overlooked.

Rob consistently highlights the importance of immediate response because in both of his cardiac arrests, rapid initiation of CPR and early use of an AED were critical to his survival and brain function preservation.

Rob acknowledged that a single CPR course taken years earlier became the difference between life and death in that moment. He stressed that while technology such as AEDs is highly important, it is the willingness and ability of people to act that ultimately determines survival. He expressed deep gratitude for his family, particularly his son, who played a direct role in saving his life, reinforcing that anyone could be in a position to save a life and that learning CPR is critical to be ready for that moment.

"I can never thank my family enough for saving my life," Rob said. "The most important thing is knowing CPR. It keeps blood flowing to the brain and heart. Take a class. Get certified. What's the cost of saving a life?"

Melody Naroleski

When I spoke with Melody Naroleski, she explained that her cardiac arrest occurred during what began as a completely ordinary workday. She has no memory of the actual collapse and instead recalls waking up much later in the hospital, being informed that she had survived a cardiac arrest.

Scan to learn more about Melody's story.

"I was at work in the city. It was just a normal day. We had just ordered lunch, and my friend had come back from a home assessment. We were sitting there talking about a movie, then the next thing I knew…"

Melody described hearing from the medical staff that she had experienced cardiac arrest as disorienting because she had no recollection of the event itself and had to rely entirely on others to piece together what happened.

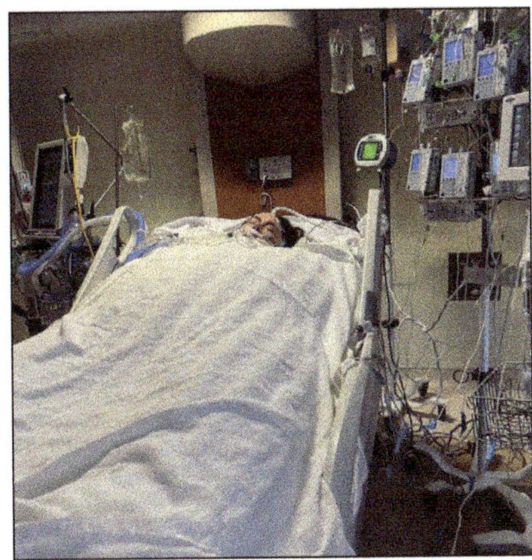
Melody in the hospital after her sudden cardiac arrest.

The people around Melody did not immediately recognize she was in distress, mistaking her unresponsiveness for joking. It quickly became clear that something was wrong when Melody stopped responding and began showing physical signs of cardiac arrest. The environment around her rapidly shifted into an emergency response, with co-workers moving furniture, calling for help, and attempting to get access to trained individuals as quickly as possible.

A critical factor in Melody's survival was the presence of a certified nursing assistant training program in the same building. "Thank God we had a CNA school upstairs. A registered nurse, Miss Teal, came down with her class and started CPR on me before EMTs even got there," Melody said, referring to the nurse as a "little angel of a woman." "If it wasn't for them, I don't know what would have happened. If this had happened at my other job in a private office, I think I would be dead."

Melody described the severity of her condition based on what she was told afterward. "My best friend was there, and he's still traumatized by it," she said. "He thought I was joking and even asked, 'Are you joking?' because I wasn't responding. They said I turned different colors, then they threw my desk aside."

Melody required multiple doses of epinephrine, was resuscitated more than once, and underwent advanced interventions, including therapeutic cooling. During her hospitalization, testing revealed no structural heart disease or blockages. Her cardiac arrest was attributed to an arrhythmia with no clearly identified cause, reinforcing the unpredictability of sudden cardiac arrest. She remained hospitalized for an extended period and ultimately had a defibrillator implanted as a precautionary measure to manage future risk. She was diagnosed with sleep apnea, which became part of her ongoing care.

Melody's recovery included both physical and emotional components. Physically, she returned to work relatively quickly and resumed many aspects of her normal routine, with ongoing follow-up care through cardiology and device monitoring.

However, Melody's emotional impact was more complex, particularly in the early stages after the event. She became acutely aware of her body and experienced fear in response to even minor sensations, stating that after the event, she wondered at every little pain, *Is this it again?*

It is important to have support systems to navigate that phase of recovery, and Melody noted that connecting with other people who experienced similar events helped her feel less isolated. She explained that prior to sharing her story publicly, only close family and friends were aware of what had happened. It took time for her to feel comfortable discussing it more openly.

Through that process, Melody recognized the value of sharing her experience to help other people understand the impact of CPR and the reality of survival. Her perspective highlights both the unpredictability of cardiac arrest and the importance of having trained people nearby who are willing to act without hesitation. "Learning CPR is important because it gives people the ability to intervene in critical moments. You just never know when it's going to come in handy," Melody said.

Michael Simpson II and His Parents, Michael Simpson Sr. and Kim Croom: In God's Hands Foundation

A fellow Ohioan, Michael Simpson Jr's story is one that shifts your understanding of what survival really means. On New Year's Day 2020, when Michael was just 18 years old, he suffered a sudden cardiac arrest while playing basketball with friends. The cardiac arrest could have ended his life instantly. Instead, it began a different kind of journey.

Scan to learn more.

"Michael was literally in God's hands," said his mother, Kim Croom.

Although help was on the way for Michael, no CPR was initiated, and although two AEDs were present, they were not used in those critical early moments. "No one knew what to do," Kim said.

When paramedics arrived, Michael had no pulse and wasn't breathing. He was resuscitated on the scene and rushed to the hospital, where he was diagnosed with an anomalous coronary artery. Mike endured multiple cardiac arrests, was placed on extracorporeal membrane oxygenation (ECMO), underwent emergency heart surgery, and faced severe complications, including anoxic brain injury, temporary blindness, and memory loss.

What followed was not just survival, but reconstruction—physically, mentally, and spiritually.

After sustaining an anoxic brain injury, Michael needed to learn how to walk, talk, and live again. Through that process, what could have remained a private struggle became something greater. His parents described the experience as traumatic and uncertain. They leaned heavily on their faith while navigating complex medical decisions and prolonged recovery during the COVID-19 pandemic.

Despite his many challenges, Michael demonstrated remarkable resilience, gradually regaining his vision, mobility, and independence through intensive rehabilitation. "You might not be where you wanted to be, but you're not where you *used* to be either," Michael said.

Michael and his family transformed their experience into purpose by founding In God's Hands Foundation, an effort grounded in education, awareness, and action. The foundation focuses on educating people on how to recognize sudden cardiac arrest, the importance of CPR, the use of AEDs, and brain injury awareness. Their work reflects a deeper understanding that survival is not just about the moment of resuscitation—rather it is about what comes after.

Today, Michael shares his story to inspire others—especially young people—while continuing therapy, community involvement, and advocacy. Michael embodies survival, faith, and growth despite life-altering adversity.

Michael's story reminds us that preparedness, immediate response, and access to CPR and AEDs are lifesaving necessities that shape outcomes long before and long after the event itself.

"I'm supposed to be dead, so anything I do is extra," Michael said.

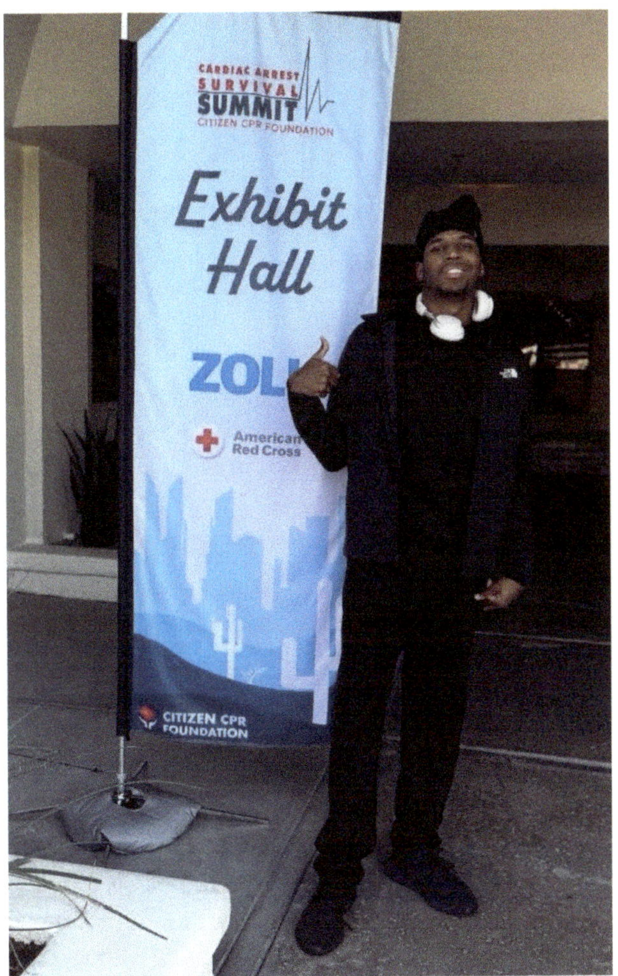

Michael Simpson II

Kim Mangine and Matthew Mangine Sr.: Matthew Mangine Jr.: One Shot Foundation

Scan to learn more about One Shot Foundation.

I became inspired by the One Shot Foundation after hearing of the Mangine family's story on a Lifesaving Summit Conference Call. Later, I met Matthew and Kim Magine at the Cardiac Arrest Survival Summit. I learned even more about their son Matthew in an even later podcast interview.

Matthew Mangine Jr. was a 16-year-old high school soccer player in Northern Kentucky. In June 2020, during a summer soccer conditioning session, he collapsed on the field.

At first, people thought Matthew had a seizure, but the collapse was later identified as sudden cardiac arrest. Emergency response began on site. An AED was present on campus; however, it was not used immediately. CPR was initiated, but reports describe delays and a lack of coordinated response in the early moments following his collapse.

Emergency medical services arrived and delivered the first AED shock 10 to 12 minutes after the initial event. “The closest AED was 250 feet away, yet it took 12 minutes to deliver the first shock. Minutes were precious, and they were lost. If a few things had gone right, we’d be having a completely different conversation about our son,” said Matt Mangine Sr.

Matthew Mangine Jr. did not survive.

Following Matthew’s death, his parents began sharing their story through national and regional media, as well as in educational and advocacy settings.

In our interview, Kim and Matthew described how their lives shifted completely after the loss of their son. They went from working traditional careers into full-time advocacy centered on sudden cardiac arrest awareness and prevention. When they reflected upon the events surrounding Matthew’s collapse, they realized that the loss of their son was not due to a lack of resources alone, but rather it was due to a breakdown in recognition, urgency, and coordinated response.

Kim and Matthew established the Matthew Mangine Jr. One Shot Foundation. Through this work, they focus on CPR education, AED access, and emergency preparedness in schools and athletic programs. They speak publicly about sudden cardiac arrest and response readiness. They stress the importance of immediate recognition of the cardiac arrest, starting CPR without hesitation, and quickly retrieving and using an AED. They advocate for removing complexity and fear from bystander response, reinforcing that perfection is not required—action is. A central theme in their approach is repetition and accessibility. Rather than relying solely on traditional certification models, they promote frequent, brief, hands-on practice through programs like “Take 10,” which aim to build muscle memory and normalize intervention, especially among younger populations.

“We also explore systemic gaps in schools and organizations, including inconsistent emergency planning, lack of follow-through after training, and over-reliance on the assumption that emergency preparedness is already in place,” Kim said. “Just because there is an emergency preparedness plan doesn’t mean people are prepared to follow it.”

The closest AED was 250 feet away, yet it took 12 minutes to deliver the first shock. Minutes were precious, and they were lost. If a few things had gone right, we’d be having a completely different conversation about our son.
—Matt Mangine Sr., Matthew’s father

The One Shot Foundation’s ultimate goal is to create a cultural shift where CPR and AED awareness are treated as basic life skills, similar to fire safety. Underlying all of their work is a strong sense of purpose shaped by personal loss—transforming frustration and grief into a mission to reduce preventable deaths and ensure other people are better prepared to act in critical moments.

“It is still a pain, an ache in my heart every day. I don’t want anyone else to go through this,” Kim said.

JJ Machnik, Laura Machnik, Trevor Hodges, and Marlana Hodges

Another story that unfolded through more than one voice for the Wellness Pulse was JJ Machnik's cardiac arrest. I Zoomed with JJ and his mother, Laura Machnik, and their family friends Trevor Hodges and his mother, Marlana Hodges.

"I'm JJ Machnik. I'm 19 years old. I survived cardiac arrest, pretty crazy, yeah," JJ introduced himself.

When Trevor was 14 years old, he saved JJ's life.

The Machnik and Hodges families had known each other for a long time through wrestling, becoming as close as family.

JJ's father had hypertrophic cardiomyopathy, which is a disease of the heart muscle that affects how well the heart pumps and can lead to serious rhythm problems. JJ and his siblings were tested for the condition because it can run in families, but his results were normal.

But two years later during a routine sports physical, further evaluation revealed that JJ did have the condition. "Our pediatrician said, 'I'm not clearing JJ for sports. He needs to go to a cardiologist,'" Laura said.

JJ's life shifted significantly because he could no longer participate in the activities that had previously defined his life. "It was a whole summer of telling him he couldn't run, couldn't ride his bike. How do you tell your ridiculously active child he can't do anything?" Laura asked.

"I went from riding around with my friends all the time to not being able to do anything. I was heartbroken. I couldn't wrestle. I couldn't play baseball. I kind of didn't really have much," JJ said.

But JJ's doctor had told him, "You could die," which while difficult to hear helped him understand the seriousness of his condition. Despite the risks, JJ was eventually cleared to participate in sporting activities with precautions, one of which included always having access to a defibrillator.

JJ carried an AED with him consistently, integrating it into his daily life. His family and community ensured that people around him were aware of his condition and prepared to respond if necessary.

> I'm 19 years old. I survived cardiac arrest, pretty crazy, yeah. I went from riding around with my friends all the time to not being able to do anything. I was heartbroken. I couldn't wrestle. I couldn't play baseball. I kind of didn't really have much.
> —JJ Machnik

This preparation extended beyond the immediate family. Their wrestling community also made adjustments, including acquiring a defibrillator to have present during events.

"We didn't want to take a chance that we couldn't get to an AED," Marlena said.

JJ has little memory of the cardiac event. He only recalls arriving at the house before losing awareness.

Marlena explained that they have wrestling mats and workout equipment in their basement, and the wrestlers are always at her house. "They're always training, working out, getting ready for tournaments," she said. "JJ and his friend Gio came over

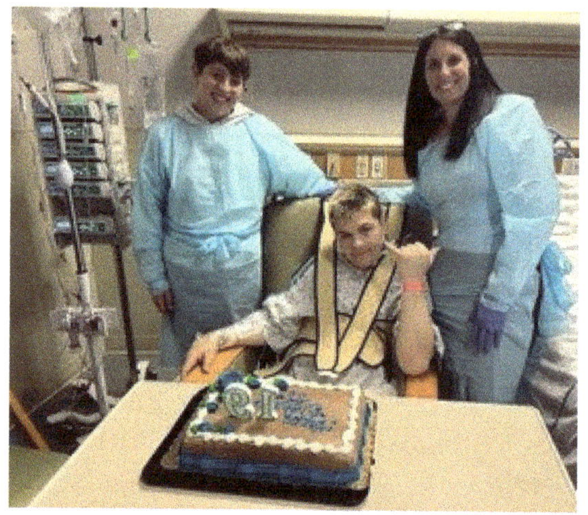

JJ Machnik's 19th birthday

that morning because they had to lose a couple pounds for a wrestling tournament they were going to that weekend. Our door's always open for the kids, so they came in, said hello, then got on the scale to weigh themselves. JJ was still a few pounds over, so he said he was gonna suit up, get his sweatshirt and sweatpants on, and go down to use the treadmill."

Next, Marlena heard a sudden noise. Immediately, she knew something was wrong, particularly given JJ's known condition. She called emergency services right away.

Marlena's daughter woke Trevor, who responded without hesitation. He ran downstairs, saw JJ was breathing at first, then stopped.

Trevor started compressions.

Gio did breaths.

"We kept going until responders got there," Trevor said.

"If Trevor did not do CPR, that child would not be here. Our story would have ended completely differently," Laura said, adding that although JJ required extensive medical intervention, including multiple resuscitations and advanced life support measures, the early CPR gave him a chance to survive and recover.

"JJ coded twice on the way to the hospital," Laura continued. "At one point, they told us that they had done everything they could. His heart was working against them. We thought that was it. But then, his heart started working again. Just like that."

The hospital phase of the story is described as unstable and uncertain, with rapid changes in JJ's condition. At times, the medical team expressed concern about his ability to recover.

Thankfully, JJ came to a turning point when his condition began to improve, leading to stabilization and eventual recovery. Laura reflected that was unpredictable, vacillating between fear and hope. "He was on ECMO. They talked about a transplant, but then suddenly, he turned around," Laura said.

JJ's recovery included both physical and emotional components. Physically, he returned to a level of functioning that surprised even the medical staff, while emotionally, he began to process the experience and its implications for his future. He reflected on the moment he left the hospital, describing how the staff acknowledged his survival, but also expressing a sense of humility.

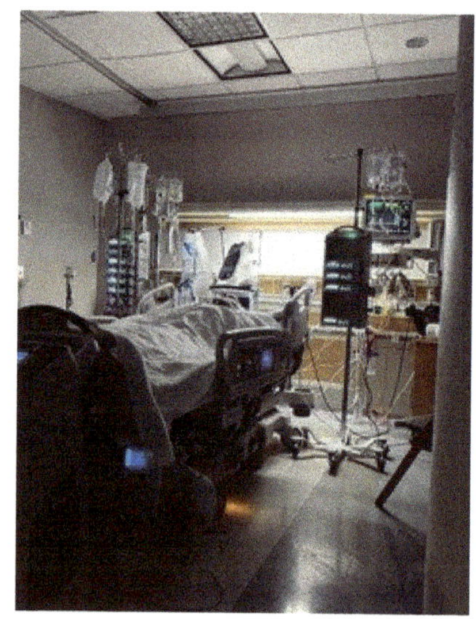

JJ in the hospital following his sudden cardiac arrest.

"I remember my birthday in the hospital. When I left, the staff lined the halls and clapped. But I felt like *they* should be the ones being applauded. I wish I could do something for them. Because they saved my life," JJ said.

JJ reflected on the broader implications of his condition, particularly in relation to the activities he once loved. He described the tension between wanting to live fully and recognizing the risks involved, acknowledging that engaging in those activities carries uncertainty. He values the quality of life those activities provide, but he also recognizes that "you don't really want to gamble your life." Today, JJ aspires to be an electrician.

Trevor remains grounded in the moment of action rather than the aftermath. He feels grateful that he could save his friend. His account emphasizes the importance of preparation and the ability to act without hesitation. Trevor's prior CPR training translated into immediate action when it was needed most.

In this family's story, multiple layers of preparedness, medical awareness, access to equipment, and trained individuals converged in a critical moment to produce a successful outcome.

Bethany Keime and Hannah Keime: HeartCharged

I had the pleasure of meeting Bethany Keime of HeartCharged at the Cardiac Arrest Survival Summit (CASS), where she was presenting an academic session with Dr. Benjamin Abella and Aubi Nemeth. These ladies are serious advocates for equality in resuscitation.

Scan to learn more about HeartCharged.

I knew Aubi from the Lifesaving Summit. She is an advocate for women, a certified registered nurse anesthesiologist (CRNA, a Basic Life Support and Advanced Cardiac Life Support instructor, amongst other things. Through Aubi and PRESTAN, I became acquainted with the HeartCharged Mission.

"Once upon a time, we were average high-school girls. Then we were diagnosed with hypertrophic cardiomyopathy (HCM), which is better than not being diagnosed but not as good as not having it," said Bethany Keime. Bethany was referring to her and her sister Hannah.

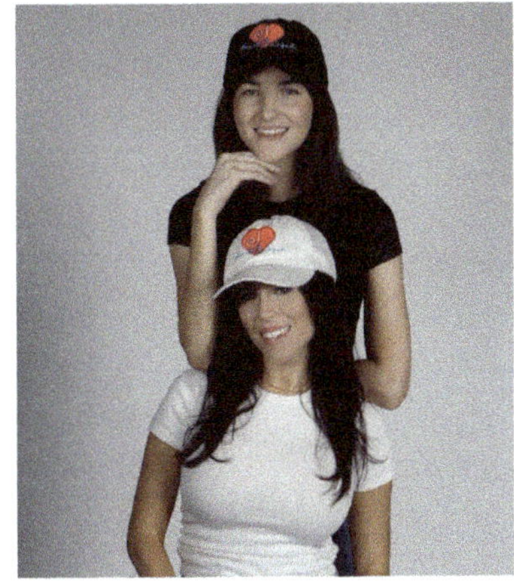

Bethany Keime and Hannah Keime

After the CASS, I caught up with the ladies of HeartCharged, and they shared their journey from diagnosis as teens to founding HeartCharged, which focuses on preventing sudden cardiac death and supporting patients through awareness, education, and advocacy.

HCM is a genetic condition and a leading cause of sudden cardiac death in young athletes. HCM causes thickening of the heart muscle, which can disrupt blood flow and lead to dangerous arrhythmias and cardiac arrest, often in young people who may otherwise appear healthy. This condition is often asymptomatic and often unidentified. Bethany and Hannah's diagnosis came through family screening.

Following their diagnosis, both sisters were placed on medication. They also made significant lifestyle adjustments to manage their heart rates and reduce the risk of dangerous arrhythmias.

"We were immediately put on medications and made lifestyle changes so that our heart rates wouldn't go up, causing our hearts to fibrillate and causing us to die," Bethany said.

As their condition progressed, those measures were no longer sufficient. Each sister received an implantable cardioverter-defibrillator (ICD), which is a device designed to detect and correct life-threatening heart rhythms.

"The device would shock our hearts if they went out of control. We are so grateful to have found out and be managing our conditions. With that gratitude, we are trying to warn the world," Bethany said.

"Our mission at Heart Charged is to end preventable deaths from undiagnosed heart conditions and sudden cardiac arrest," Hannah said. Their work emphasizes early detection, preparedness in emergencies, and access to lifesaving interventions, such as CPR and defibrillation.

"Childhood deaths from undiagnosed heart conditions are preventable. Because we were screened and it saved our lives, we want *all* children to have the heart screenings they need. But we also need people prepared to act in an emergency," Bethany said.

The sisters' efforts extended into presentations and collaborations across medical, advocacy, and community spaces, including engagements with organizations such as the American Heart Association, Global Heart Hub, and WomenHeart. They also participate in conferences, patient engagement summits, and school-based education programs.

"Because we had each other to share the day-to-day dealings with our conditions, we want others to connect. Because our hearts still quiver, we want others to know we walk on without surety. Because our souls still find joy, we want others to smile loudly," Bethany said.

"We were very lucky that we had each other through our diagnosis. That's really the foundation of Heart Charged: Knowing that you're not alone," Hannah said.

Bethany and Hannah contributed to awareness through media and creative projects, including podcasts, interviews, social campaigns, and short films on living with HCM and invisible disability. Their work focuses on disparities in cardiac arrest response, youth education in CPR and AED use, and community-based training efforts designed to increase confidence and action during emergencies.

They are also passionate about critical issues like misdiagnosis, lack of symptom recognition, gender disparities in CPR response, and the emotional toll of living with a life-threatening condition. Through personal experiences, including surviving cardiac arrest and navigating life with implantable defibrillators, they emphasize the importance of community, mental health support, and empowering everyday people to act—whether by recognizing symptoms, getting screened, or performing CPR without hesitation.

Martha Lopez-Anderson: Parent Heart Watch

Scan to learn more about Parent Heart Watch.

I met Martha Lopez-Anderson of Parent Heart Watch at the Lifesaving Summit in 2024. I also heard her speak and was struck by the depth of her message. She spoke about Parent Heart Watch and the Call, Push, Shock campaign. When her son Sean Anderson was 10 years old, he collapsed while rollerblading outside his home. It was later discovered he had suffered sudden cardiac arrest. There had been no prior warning signs, and his condition had gone undetected. According to the Parent Heart Watch website, people who witnessed his collapse thought he was having a seizure.

> I could not understand how my seemingly healthy child could suddenly collapse and die.
> —Martha Lopez-Anderson

Sean received CPR, but an AED was not immediately available. It took approximately 10 minutes for one to arrive.

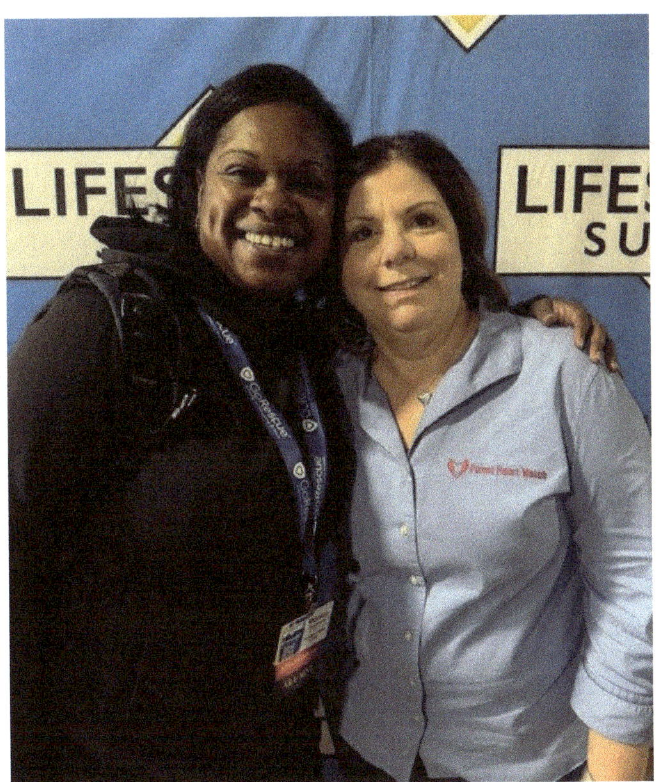

Martha Lopez-Anderson and me

Sean did not survive.

Martha described the experience as unexpected. Sean appeared to be healthy. "I could not understand how my seemingly healthy child could suddenly collapse and die," she said.

Following Sean's death, Martha and her husband began working in the space of sudden cardiac arrest awareness. They founded an organization called Saving Young Hearts that focused on youth heart screenings and education. That organization operated for about 15 years

Over time, Martha's work expanded into national advocacy through Parent Heart Watch, where she is currently Executive Director. Parent Heart Watch is a national organization dedicated to protecting children and young adults from sudden cardiac arrest and preventable sudden cardiac death through education and advocacy. The organization was founded by parents who lost children to sudden cardiac arrest and came together to better understand what had happened and how similar outcomes could be prevented. It has since grown into a nationwide network that includes families, survivors, medical professionals, and advocates working to improve both prevention and emergency response in youth settings.

Their work includes promoting heart screenings to identify underlying conditions, expanding access to AEDs, and supporting CPR and emergency response training in schools and communities. To date, Parent Heart Watch has contributed to more than 1.3 million youth

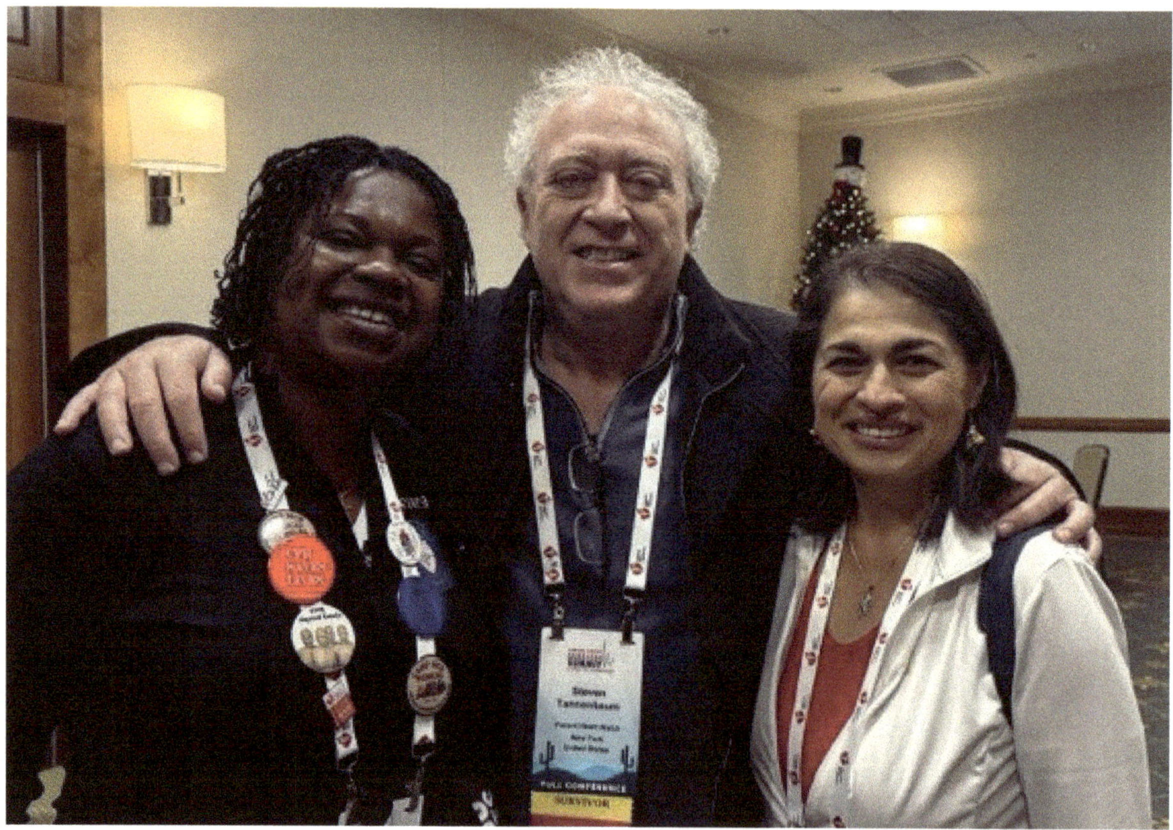

Steven Tannenbaum and me

heart screenings, trained over 950,000 individuals in CPR and AED use, and helped place more than 13,000 AEDs in communities.

The organization is also a collaborator in national awareness efforts such as the Call-Push-Shock campaign, which was launched in partnership with the Sudden Cardiac Arrest Foundation to encourage immediate recognition of cardiac arrest, initiation of CPR, and use of an AED. Parent Heart Watch's work centers on increasing preparedness and response in the moments where early action can influence survival.

I ran into Steven Tannenbaum of Parent Heart Watch in Phoenix at the CASS. Steve was passionate about educating the public on the fact that 23,000 die each year from cardiac arrest. He wants the public to know that Parent Heart Watch is a tremendous advocate of primary prevention, which includes heart screening (EKGs) to detect abnormalities that aren't regularly performed on healthy children. Parent Heart Watch is making gains and getting children screened.

I've been honored to present these stories of people affected by sudden cardiac arrest. These accounts were gathered by various means—through conversations, brief exchanges, and shared moments with individuals and families. Some were shared in depth, others more briefly, but each reflects a moment that did not last long, even if its impact did. The details vary. The settings change. The outcomes are not the same.

For all of the people involved, critical recovery followed. Often, ongoing adjustments were needed to adapt to what had happened both physically and emotionally. What carries forward is not only what happened, but what *continues* because of it.

Across these stories, something else takes shape: the awareness of how much difference a single response can make. The next sudden cardiac arrest could happen anywhere, to anyone. ***Hopefully, a response will come from someone nearby who chose to be ready.***

Chapter 12: One World, One Beat

When I began this journey of unraveling the origins of CPR, I had a hunch that CPR was born out of desperation. I was right.

What has not changed in human history is that sudden cardiac arrest happens everywhere, without warning and without time to prepare in the moment. What *has* changed is how the world responds to it. Thanks to global research, shared guidelines, and ongoing collaboration, we now have a clearer understanding of what saves lives: early recognition, immediate CPR, and access to defibrillation.

But that knowledge alone is not enough. When life hangs in the balance, it still depends on whether someone is present, prepared, and willing to act when it matters most.

As a passionate advocate for CPR and AED education, creating this book was a labor of love. From my years as a nurse and CPR instructor, building and growing People's Choice CPR, The Wellness Pulse, and researching and writing this book, I gained so much knowledge and inspiration that I wanted to share it—to help inform and inspire other people across the globe, having this same human experience, to be present, prepared, and willing to act.

I hope this book will inspire you to go beyond by interacting with the QR codes for the podcast episodes that expand the stories on these pages. Please visit the websites of those organizations I have mentioned. Learn more. Get involved more. Be more.

I hope that you understand how important we all can be in the chain of survival. Seconds feel small, until they are everything.

Learn CPR. Practice it. Stay ready.

Be part of the rhythm that keeps someone here.

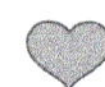

TIMELINE

Biblical Breath of Life

5500-4000 BC Genesis "God breathed Life" into man, "And the LORD God formed man of the dust of the ground, and breathed into his nostrils the breath of life; and man became a living soul."—Genesis 2:7 (KJV). The idea that life could be given through breath would later echo in human attempts to restore it—turning a divine act into a clinical pursuit.

This passage introduced a powerful early association between breath and life, positioning breath as the moment life begins, describing life not as an inherent human function, but as something imparted. The act of God breathing into man established breath as the defining threshold between lifeless matter and a living being. This concept echoed forward into resuscitation practices, where restoring breath became synonymous with restoring life. Long before formal medicine, this idea laid a philosophical foundation that would later manifest in lifesaving techniques centered around airway and ventilation.

870 BC 1st Kings Elijah resuscitated a Phoenician boy in the city of Zarephath. 1 Kings 17:17-24. "And he stretched himself upon the child three times, and cried unto the LORD, and said, O LORD my God, I pray thee, let this child's soul come into him again. And the LORD heard the voice of Elijah; and the soul of the child came into him again and he revived."

In Zarephath, Elijah responded to the death of a child not with passive mourning, but with action—stretching himself over the body repeatedly while calling for the return of life. This moment stands as one of the earliest depictions of deliberate human intervention in death, where physical effort and faith intersect in an attempt to revive the lifeless.

This account represented one of the earliest recorded resuscitation attempts, combining physical intervention with spiritual invocation. The act reflected an early belief that life could be called back—not only through prayer, but through intentional physical intervention. The act of laying body-to-body suggests an intuitive understanding that life could be restored through physical contact, possibly facilitating warmth, stimulation, and the transfer of breath.

This passage is often cited as one of the earliest descriptions of hands-on resuscitative effort. Elijah's actions—placing himself over the child and repeating the act—demonstrated an early, non-formalized approach to resuscitation. While not described in anatomical terms, the positioning implies chest-to-chest contact and potential airway alignment, paralleling later concepts of ventilation and circulation support. This event marked a transition from breath as a divine gift to breath as something that could be actively restored.

850-840 BC Elisha did mouth-to-mouth in Shunem in ancient Israel. 2 Kings 4:32-35, "And he went up, and lay upon the child, and put his mouth upon his mouth, and his eyes upon his eyes, and his hands upon his hands, and he stretched himself upon the child; and the flesh of the child waxed warm."

Elisha's actions were described with a level of precision that closely parallels core principles seen in modern CPR. By placing his mouth on the child's mouth, he established a direct airway connection, suggesting an early form of assisted breathing. His full-body alignment—eyes to eyes and hands to hands—indicates intentional positioning, which in modern terms supports airway control, chest alignment, and overall physiologic support. The response unfolded in recognizable stages: The child's body begins to warm, reflecting a return of circulation or metabolic activity; Elisha then repeats the intervention, demonstrating persistence rather than a single attempt; and finally, the child exhibits clear signs of life, marked by sneezing and revival.

This sequence mirrors the fundamental structure of resuscitation today—airway, breathing, repeated effort, and observable response—positioning this account as one of the earliest depictions of a deliberate, hands-on attempt to restore life through what would eventually evolve into organized resuscitative practice.

160-120 AD Greek and Roman physicians, including Galen, explored early concepts of artificial respiration, documenting methods of inflating the lungs using devices such as bellows or reeds inserted into the airway. These approaches reflected a growing anatomical understanding that air movement was essential to sustaining life. While not formalized into standardized practice, these efforts represent some of the earliest recorded attempts to mechanically support breathing in cases of asphyxia or drowning. Observations of chest movement and the effects of air insufflation began to shift resuscitation from purely philosophical or spiritual interpretations toward anatomical and physiological experimentation.

300-700 In various African Christian healing traditions, including those associated with the Kingdom of Aksum, care for the unresponsive included both spiritual and physical elements. Practitioners assessed whether breathing had ceased and offered prayers specifically calling for the return of breath. Physical interventions—such as warming the body, positioning, and tactile stimulation—were used alongside these prayers.

In regions such as Nubia and Kush, as well as parts of West Africa, healing practices emphasized restoring vitality through warmth, oils, and physical stimulation—often accompanied by spiritual invocation. While much of this knowledge was likely transmitted orally, these approaches reflected a continued recognition that breath, warmth, and physical responsiveness were central indicators of life, blending spiritual belief with practical observation. Early interpretations of breath as life began to evolve into attempts to understand and manipulate breathing through physical and mechanical means.

265-420 Jin Dynasty, Ge Hong wrote *Baopuzi* in 300 AD. He described methods aimed at restoring breathing in people who appeared lifeless, particularly in cases such as drowning or unconscious victims to restore breathing. He emphasized death, warmth, and continued effort. (The title *Baopuzi* was hard to translate. It's the idea is that we are holding onto life at the most basic level. It's complicated to put into words and is often things like "The master who embraces simplicity" or "The philosopher who holds the uncharted block." According to my research, these things mean they are focused on preserving life, which include breathing and revival.)

600-650 Ahrun of Alexandria, a Christian physician, wrote a medical compendium focusing on practical care. The original work was in Syriac, but it was later translated into Arabic and came to be utilized by early Islamic physicians. He contributed to the preservation and transmission of Greco-Roman medical knowledge, particularly Galen, allowing for a bridge of information from the previous Christian medical practices into what was known as the Islamic Golden age.

610 Sui Dynasty, *Zhubing Yuanhou Lun (Treatise on the Origins and Symptoms of Disease),* authored by Chao Yuanfang blatantly discussed resuscitation after drowning or hanging. It outlined practical steps aimed at restoring breathing, including positioning the body, relieving airway obstruction, and applying physical stimulation. The emphasis on continued effort and observation reflected an emerging understanding that revival was a process rather than an immediate event.

In contrast to earlier methods that were rooted primarily in spiritual or symbolic action, these descriptions presented resuscitation as a repeatable and teachable response grounded in physical intervention. This work represented a shift toward systematized medical thinking, where restoring breath became part of a broader framework of diagnosis, intervention, and expected response.

618-907 The Tang Dynasty produced more formalized medical trainings, clearer instructions with more procedural detail, and a desire for practical techniques. Texts by Sun Simiao, also known as the "King of Medicine" in China, included directions for reviving people from hanging, drowning, or suffocation. He described clearing the airway, restoring breathing by blowing air into the lungs to assist ventilation, and continuing the efforts even when the person appeared dead. This era began to seriously use aids for ventilation like reeds, tubes, and hollow devices. Effectiveness, hygiene, and modesty might have been contributing motivators.

750-1258 Islamic Golden Age, a time in which airway, breathing, and revival became increasingly procedural, written, taught, and disseminated. Medical knowledge was actively preserved, translated, and expanded upon, particularly through organized efforts to translate Greek works—such as those of Galen and Hippocrates—into Arabic.

These texts were not only preserved but critically studied, corrected, and built upon, forming the foundation of a more structured and evidence-informed medical system. Institutions known as bimaristans functioned as early hospitals, serving as centers for both patient care and medical education. Within these settings, physicians emphasized clinical observation, documentation, and repeatable treatment approaches.

Conditions such as asphyxia, suffocation, and drowning were increasingly recognized as treatable medical emergencies rather than irreversible events. Interventions focused on restoring breathing through positioning, airway clearance, stimulation, and in some cases assisted ventilation using rudimentary tools such as reeds or tubes. These practices reflected a growing understanding that sustaining or restoring airflow was central to preserving life.

This era marked a transition from isolated acts of revival to a more organized medical responsibility where restoring breath became part of a broader clinical framework supported by teaching, written instruction, and institutional practice. Knowledge was no longer confined to individual practitioners, but it was systematically recorded, taught, and disseminated across regions, including Persia, Syria, and Egypt. This created a medical system where revival became standard medical duty, not merely an exception.

865-925 In Persia (Iran), Al-Razi (Rhazes) was the head physician of major hospitals referred to as bimaristans. He wrote on airway obstruction, asphyxia, and drowning. He emphasized clinical observation over theory, contributing to the growing recognition that breathing failure was a treatable medical crisis.

980-1037 In Persia, Avicenna (Ibn Sina) authored *Canon of Medicine*, depicting respiratory physiology, suffocation, and near-deaths. He emphasized careful assessment and intervention before declaring death.. Breath was identified as central to sustaining and restoring life.

1213-1288 In Syria/Egypt, Ibn al-Nafis described pulmonary circulation, identifying that blood passes through the lungs before returning to the heart and that the lungs were increasingly recognized as essential to life.

It is important to note that things got a little sketchy after this, as far as CPR progression. The world was limited in communication at that time. Works that were discovered in Islamic areas were often not translated into other languages, and the same in reverse. Works that were developed in Arabic, Chinese, and European contexts were inaccessible to each other. Medical advances that were happening around the world were not equal and not equally shared.

Therefore, many scholars and researchers were led to test or retest things that had already been proven in different areas of the world or during different time frames. All in all, that resulted in stagnation and/or regression of CPR advancements.

1258 The fall of Baghdad in 1258 represented a political collapse and a significant disruption in the preservation and advancement of medical knowledge. Baghdad was a major center of scholarship within the Abbasid Caliphate, and as such it housed extensive libraries, hospitals, and educational institutions that supported the translation, study, and practice of medicine. When Mongol forces, led by Hulagu Khan, overtook the city during the rule of Al-Musta'sim, much of this infrastructure was destroyed.

Contemporary accounts describe the loss of manuscripts on a massive scale—sometimes illustrated by reports of the Tigris River darkened with ink—capturing the magnitude of intellectual loss, whether interpreted literally or symbolically.

The destruction of bimaristans, libraries, and scholarly networks disrupted systems that had supported medical education, documentation, and clinical practice. This event slowed the momentum of structured medical advancement in the region, and it marked a significant interruption in the continuity of knowledge that had been developing for centuries. Although not all of the knowledge immediately vanished, the momentum dissipated. Because there was no European hospital system equivalent, no emergency care systems similar to the bimaristans, and no experimental medicine research, future scientists had to rediscover and revisit topics.

1300-1500s Europe entered an era where progress in systematic resuscitation techniques slowed. Religious doctrine often overrode scientific experimentation, which led to no advancement in systematic revival techniques. However, the idea that restoration of breathing restored life did not disappear.

1493-1541 Paracelsus, a Swiss physician, challenged traditional reliance on ancient authorities and emphasized observation and hands-on treatment. Early efforts to restore breathing included the use of mechanical means such as bellows to force air into the lungs—an approach that reflected growing recognition of the importance of airflow in sustaining life. This was an early attempt at instrumental artificial respiration—conceptually *huge,* albeit crude.

During this period, medicine began to shift toward experimentation and direct intervention. These methods were not yet standardized, but they represented an important conceptual step toward artificial respiration, where breathing was no longer only observed but actively manipulated in attempts to preserve life.

1420-1480 Burhān al-Dīn al-Kirmānī described Ghashy/Ghāshī *(ghashy)*, a condition characterized by sudden loss of consciousness, weak or absent pulse, and impaired breathing—likely corresponding to syncope or collapse. Rather than a single disease, it was understood as a clinical state requiring response.

Treatment approaches focused on restoring responsiveness through physical stimulation, warming, and positioning. Techniques included vigorous rubbing of the chest and limbs, application of warm compresses, and using aromatic stimulants such as camphor or vinegar to provoke breathing. Inhalants like ambergris, camphor, cardamom, cinnamon, musk, or vinegar smoke or vapors were blown or bellowed into the nostrils.

Positioning strategies were also employed, including lowering the head or placing the person laterally. These methods reflected an evolving recognition that collapse and apparent lifelessness could be reversible and that physical intervention could influence breathing and circulation.

The manuscripts were written in Persian, thus preventing the information from being shared globally. However, the information would lend to European rediscovery.

1600-1700s The inversion method involved suspending an unconscious, typically drowning victim often by their ankles in an attempt to expel water and stimulate breathing. This was done typically in Europe and colonial environments. It was recommended in early drowning manuals and folklore medicine.

Different explanations made this a desirable emergency response: Belief that the stimulation might shock the body, that gravity or inversion could restore life because the vital spirits were believed to be housed in the head and the inversion could restart the life force, or simply the belief that the draining of the water would restore breathing.

1667 Robert Hooke demonstrated that fresh air, not merely movement of the chest, was essential to sustaining life.

1732 Scottish Surgeon William A. Tossach used mouth-to-mouth to resuscitate James Blair, a coal miner in Alloa, Scotland. He is recorded as being dead for 30 to 45 minutes. His resuscitation was witnessed by a crowd of nearly 400 people. He returned to work a few days later.

This is considered to be one of the earliest well-documented successful uses of mouth-to-mouth resuscitation in the modern era. Dr. Tossach published an account of this occurrence in 1744.

1767 This year marked the first organized effort to respond to sudden death by a group of Amsterdam citizens, the Society for the Recovery of Drowned Persons. Their recommendations included mouth-to-mouth, warming of the victim, water expulsion efforts via inversion, manual pressure applied to the abdomen, and stimulation by rectal fumigation with tobacco smoke and bloodletting. They are credited with saving 150 lives within four years.

1769 Hamburg, Germany, passed an ordinance allowing notices in church describing rescue methods for people who were drowned, frozen, strangled, or overcome by noxious gases.

1773 Organizations similar to the Society for the Recovery of Drowned Persons were created in Hamburg, Milan, Paris, Padua, Venice, and Vienna.

1774 The Royal Humane Society was founded in London, England—the world's first known organized resuscitation organization. Their mission was simple: to restore life to people apparently drowned or dead. They offered rewards for rescuers, public instruction and trainings, and stationed equipment along rivers.

This was also the first known public emergency response system. Their recommended instruction included mouth-to-mouth, (ironically, this fell out of use and resurfaced), bellows ventilation (this was most likely inspired by Paracelsus's experimental approach to artificial respiration, but it also increased lung injuries due to excessive pressure), abdominal and chest manipulation (rolling the body, pressing on the abdomen, raising the arms), warming, and stimulation (alcohol or stimulants, blankets, hot bricks, or rubbing the body). They were big proponents of the Tobacco Smoke Enema and said kits.

1803 The Russian Method, also referred to as the Barrel-Rolling method or Rolling method, was used by the Russian empire—a technique based on rolling the victim on a barrel to force air into and out of the lungs. The thought was that expanding the chest and abdomen would provoke breathing.

1812 In the Trotting Horse Method, the victim was placed across a horse's back, and the horse was instructed to trot or walk, causing the rhythmic body movement. This forced air in and out, in an attempt to stimulate breathing through rhythmic compression and expansion. The horse was thus serving as a living ventilation machine—a whole different spin on equine therapy!

1856 In the United Kingdom. a manual artificial respiration technique called the Hall Method, named for the physiologist Marshall Hall, not to be confused with his grandson, the musician. This might have also been cited as the Ready Method because it was meant to be performed immediately on drowning victims.

The victim would be placed prone to encourage water and any bodily fluids to be expelled. Then the victim would be placed onto their side and back again repeatedly. These movements created chest and abdomen compression, forcing air out, and chest expansion, where air would flow in, creating alternating compression and expansion of the chest to encourage airflow when on their side or placed in a supine fashion. These movements were repeated 12 to 15 rolls per minute.

1858 In the United Kingdom, the Silvester's Method was developed by Henry Robert Silvester, a manual technique of moving the victim's arms to expand and compress the chest to stimulate breathing.

1869 The Howard Method was formulated by Edward Howard, an American physician. This was one of the first known attempts to use the body's mechanics to stimulate breathing. The victim would be laid on their back (supine) with their head elevated slightly and the chest and abdomen exposed. The rescuer would then press downward on the upper (epigastric) region of the abdomen. Air was expelled from the lung due to the diaphragm being pushed upward. The diaphragm naturally returned to its resting position and air flowed passively into the lungs. This was repeated 10 to 15 times per minute. Howard emphasized diaphragm displacement and abdominal pressure's role in ventilation. Schafer and Holger Nielsen would draw from this, and later manual ventilation methods would incorporate similar concepts of external pressure and chest movement.

1883 *Journal of the American Medical Association*, a peer-reviewed clinical medicine, research, public health and policy journal, was created as part of a broader effort by the American Medical Association to organize and professionalize medicine in the United States. Goals were to improve communication between physicians, elevate medical standards, and distribute clinical knowledge more consistently. What began as a professional publication gradually evolved into a major force in global medicine, shaping how research, clinical practices, and eventually emergency care and resuscitation science were shared and validated. It is one of the most influential medical journals in the world.

1891 In Hamburg, Germany, Friedrich Maass published research stating that rhythmic pressure on the chest could circulate blood throughout the body and restart circulation during cardiac failure. His research included animal and human experimentation, which was normal for the time. He documented one of the earliest uses of closed-chest cardiac massage in humans. This was almost 70 years before the development of what we know as CPR. He revived a patient using external pressure to the chest versus utilizing surgical intervention. Basically, blood can be pumped through the body by pressing hard enough on the chest. His work went largely unnoticed because it was published in German, but he clearly was ahead of his time.

1903 In the United Kingdom, the Schafer Method, also known as the Prone Pressure Method, was developed by Edward Albert Schafer. The victim was laid face down with their head turned to the side to keep the airway open. The rescuer kneeled over the victim's hips and firmly pressed on the flank, applying rhythmic pressure to the lower back and rib area for two to three seconds. This was repeated about 12 times per minute. This method was adopted by major organizations such as the Boy Scouts, the British Army, the Red Cross, and other lifesaving societies.

1932 The Holger Nielsen Technique was created in Denmark by Holger Nielsen, a prone-position that combined arm lifting to draw air in and back pressure to force air out. This method merged concepts from Silvester and Schafer into one system. This became one of the most widely adopted manual artificial respiration methods prior to modern CPR. Because this intervention avoided direct mouth contact, it became widely adopted by military organizations, Red Cross societies, scouts, and lifesaving groups prior to the re-emergence of mouth-to-mouth resuscitation. The method reflected an increasing effort to standardize and teach repeatable approaches to artificial respiration before the development of modern CPR. The Holger Nielsen method became popular partly because mouth-to-mouth breathing temporarily lost favor, only to later return and prove more effective scientifically.

1947 Dr. Claude S. Beck of Cleveland, Ohio, performed the first successful human defibrillation during open chest cardiac surgery on a 14-year-old boy at Case Western Reserve University in Cleveland, Ohio. His work helped lay the foundation for modern defibrillation and cardiac resuscitation practices. Cleveland hospitals in the 1940s and 1950s helped refine cardiac arrest protocols, proving that sudden cardiac arrest could be survived.

1954 Dr. James O. Elam of Arkansas and Buffalo, New York, an anesthesiologist, demonstrated that positive pressure ventilation (mouth-to-mouth), was not only effective but superior to previously used manual artificial respiration practices in laboratory settings. He would later partner with Dr. Peter Safar to promote rescue breathing as a viable lifesaving technique.

1956 Dr. Paul M. Zoll of Boston, Massachusetts, developed and demonstrated external defibrillation. He also helped pioneer the way in external cardiac pacing for complete heart block, using electrical impulses through the chest wall to stimulate heartbeats. These findings became the ancestors to transcutaneous pacing and implanted pacemakers.

1956 Dr. Peter Safar was born in Vienna, Austria. He was formally trained as an anesthesiologist and immigrated to the United States and was primarily based out of Pittsburgh, Pennsylvania. He is often referred to as one of the fathers of modern CPR. He worked with Dr. Elam to expand upon his work and initiate a system refining airway techniques such as the head-tilt chin lift, developed the ABC sequence, which remained the foundational in resuscitation training for at least 50 years. He integrated Kouwenhoven's chest compressions with mouth-to-mouth breathing and helped establish the framework of modern-day CPR. He created and collaborated with the creation of training protocols and global CPR standards. These developments contributed significantly to the growth of modern emergency medicine and resuscitation science.

1957 The American Heart Association began formally supporting emerging resuscitation science and cardiovascular emergency education, disseminating research on rescue breathing and cardiac revival into broader medical awareness. As evidence surrounding mouth-to-mouth ventilation and coordinated resuscitative care increased, the organization played an expanding role in the dissemination of lifesaving practices that would later contribute to standardized CPR training and emergency cardiovascular care programs.

1958 Dr. James Elam and Dr. Peter Safar published studies in the *New England Journal of Medicine* supporting the integration of rescue breathing with external chest compression concepts in resuscitation efforts. Their work helped establish mouth-to-mouth ventilation as a scientifically validated, lifesaving intervention and accelerated the movement toward coordinated modern CPR practices.

1960 At Johns Hopkins University, Dr. William Kouwenhoven, Dr. James Jude, and Guy Knickerbocker demonstrated that rhythmic external chest compressions could generate enough circulation to sustain life during cardiac arrest. Their research showed that effective blood flow could be produced without surgically opening the chest, establishing closed-chest cardiac massage as a viable resuscitative intervention. Combined with emerging rescue breathing techniques, these findings became foundational to the development of contemporary CPR.

1960 Norwegian toy maker and entrepreneur Asmund Laerdal partnered with Dr. Peter Safar, Dr. James Elam, and other resuscitation pioneers to help create Resusci Anne, the first widely used CPR training manikin. Designed to give learners a realistic way to practice mouth-to-mouth ventilation and chest compressions, Resusci Anne transformed CPR from a medical concept into a teachable public skill. The manikin helped make standardized, hands-on CPR training possible for both healthcare providers and lay rescuers.

1963 Dr. Eugene Nagel helped pioneer mobile coronary care through the development of Miami's Rescue 1 program, an early advanced cardiac response system that brought physician-guided emergency heart care into the prehospital setting. Rescue 1 utilized radio telemetry to transmit electrocardiogram (ECG) data from the field to hospitals, allowing physicians to advise treatment before the patient arrived. The program demonstrated that rapid cardiac intervention outside the hospital could improve survival and helped lay the foundation for modern paramedic systems, mobile intensive care units, and advanced prehospital cardiac life support.

1965 Dr. Frank Pantridge and Dr. John Geddes developed the world's first mobile coronary care unit in Belfast, Northern Ireland, bringing advanced cardiac treatment directly into the prehospital setting. Their ambulance-based system used portable defibrillation equipment and cardiac monitoring technology to treat patients experiencing acute myocardial infarction and sudden cardiac arrest before arrival at the hospital. Often referred to as the Father of Emergency Medicine, Dr. Pantridge helped demonstrate that rapid cardiac intervention in the field could significantly improve survival, laying the foundation for contemporary paramedic systems, mobile intensive care units, and modern prehospital cardiac care.

1966 The National Academy of Sciences and National Research Council published *Accidental Death and Disability: The Neglected Disease of Modern Society*, a landmark report exposing major deficiencies in emergency medical care throughout the United States. The report criticized inconsistent ambulance services, inadequate training, poor communication systems, and the lack of standardized emergency treatment for trauma and cardiac emergencies. Often referred to as the White Paper of EMS, it became a major catalyst for the development of organized emergency medical services, paramedic programs, standardized CPR training, and modern prehospital emergency care.

In response to the growing urgency surrounding resuscitation and emergency response, the National Academy of Sciences–National Research Council also convened the Conference on Cardiopulmonary Resuscitation in 1966. Representatives from more than 30 national organizations gathered to evaluate emerging CPR science and establish recommendations for instruction, performance, and retraining. The conference helped move CPR toward greater national consistency and accelerated the formalization of resuscitation education in both healthcare and community settings.

1967 The Freedom House Ambulance Service was established in Pittsburgh, Pennsylvania, becoming one of the first professionally trained paramedic ambulance services in the United States. Staffed primarily by African-American men and women from Pittsburgh's Hill District, the program was developed through collaboration between Dr. Peter Safar, Dr. Nancy Caroline, and community leaders to provide advanced prehospital emergency care in underserved areas.

Freedom House paramedics received rigorous medical training far beyond the standard ambulance attendants of the era, including airway management, CPR, oxygen administration, cardiac emergency response, and advanced lifesaving interventions. The success of the program helped demonstrate that highly trained prehospital providers could significantly improve emergency care outcomes and laid important groundwork for the development of modern paramedic systems nationwide.

1969-1972 Dr. Leonard Cobb, an American cardiologist and resuscitation researcher based in Seattle, Washington, helped launch one of the world's first large-scale community CPR training initiatives. Alongside Seattle Fire Chief Gordon Vickery and physicians associated with Harborview Medical Center, Dr. Cobb helped develop Medic One, a specialized paramedic response system designed to provide advanced cardiac care before patients reached the hospital, and Medic Two, a program focused on teaching CPR to ordinary community members so bystanders could begin lifesaving care immediately during cardiac emergencies.

Seattle Heart Watch also emerged during this period, collecting data on cardiac arrests, emergency response times, CPR performance, and survival outcomes to help improve resuscitation practices and out-of-hospital cardiac arrest survival rates. Together, these programs became internationally influential models for coordinated emergency medical response and widespread public CPR education.

1960s-1970s The American Heart Association (AHA), the American Red Cross, the National Academy of Sciences, and other organizations endorsed CPR, and the American Red Cross began funding CPR research. By 1966, the AHA helped present national CPR conferences. By the 1970s, the AHA developed standardized ACLS and BLS courses.

1972 Portable defibrillation and mobile coronary care gained increased public attention following cardiac emergencies involving former United States President Lyndon B. Johnson. Advancements pioneered by Dr. Frank Pantridge and colleagues in Belfast, Northern Ireland, demonstrated that cardiac monitoring and defibrillation technology could be transported directly to patients outside the hospital setting. These developments helped validate the growing importance of rapid prehospital cardiac intervention and influenced the evolution of mobile intensive care units, paramedic response systems, and contemporary emergency cardiac care.

1973 Federal Funding for EMS The Emergency Medical Services Systems Act of 1973 helped make federal funding available for the development of organized emergency medical services throughout the United States. By establishing national support and grant structures for EMS programs, the legislation allowed states, hospitals, and regional systems to obtain resources for ambulance services, paramedic training, communication networks, trauma care, and coordinated prehospital emergency response. Federal involvement helped move EMS from scattered local initiatives toward a more standardized national emergency care infrastructure.

1974 The American Heart Association published formal standards for cardiopulmonary resuscitation (CPR) and emergency cardiac care, helping establish greater national consistency in CPR instruction, performance, and training. These guidelines brought together evolving research in chest compressions, rescue breathing, cardiac monitoring, and emergency response into a more standardized framework for healthcare providers and trained rescuers. The publication helped strengthen CPR education programs and further advanced the development of organized emergency cardiac care systems throughout the United States.

1974–1975 The American Heart Association introduced Advanced Cardiac Life Support (ACLS), expanding resuscitation training beyond basic CPR to include advanced airway management, cardiac rhythm recognition, defibrillation, medications, and coordinated emergency cardiac care. Emerging from national conferences on cardiopulmonary resuscitation and emergency cardiac care during the early 1970s, ACLS helped create a more organized and standardized approach to advanced resuscitation training for healthcare professionals. The program built upon decades of foundational work in chest compressions, rescue breathing, cardiac monitoring, defibrillation, and emergency response developed by pioneers including Dr. Leonard Cobb, Dr. James Jude, Dr. William Kouwenhoven, Dr. Peter Safar, and many others involved in the evolution of contemporary resuscitation science.

1977 American Safety and Health Institute (ASHI) was established in Eugene, Oregon by Ralph E. Haig, educators, and occupational safety professionals seeking to expand practical emergency care and safety education. ASHI became an important provider of CPR, first aid, and workplace safety training programs and would later evolve into part of the Health & Safety Institute (HSI).

1978 Physio-Control, introduced the LIFEPACK 1, one of the first portable defibrillator and cardiac monitoring systems designed for prehospital emergency care. Building upon earlier work in defibrillation and mobile coronary care, the device helped expand advanced cardiac treatment into ambulances and field response systems, contributing to the evolution of modern portable defibrillation and public-access AED technology.

1979 The U.S. Surgeon General's Office launched the Healthy People Initiative with involvement from the U.S. Department of Health, Education, and Welfare and the U.S. Public Health Service. The initiative focused on improving national public health through prevention, education, and community health goals, helping increase awareness surrounding heart disease, emergency response, CPR education, and public health preparedness throughout the United States.

1979 The National Conference on Standards for Cardiopulmonary Resuscitation (CPR) and Emergency Cardiac Care (ECC) was held to update and improve CPR and emergency heart care guidelines as CPR training, paramedic programs, and emergency medical systems continued to grow across the United States. Building upon earlier CPR conferences and new research from the 1960s and 1970s, the conference helped create more consistent CPR training, emergency response practices, and advanced cardiac care standards for healthcare workers and trained rescuers.

1980 The Conference on CPR was held at Baylor University in Houston, Texas. Over time, the concepts and collaborative efforts surrounding these meetings would contribute to what later became the Cardiac Arrest Survival Summit. This conference was somewhat unusual for its time because it focused heavily on bystanders, community CPR training, dispatcher-assisted CPR, and public access to AEDs.

1985 Dr. Michael "Mickey" Eisenberg, an American emergency physician and public health researcher based in Seattle, Washington, helped expand Seattle's emergency cardiac care system and advanced research surrounding sudden cardiac arrest survival. He helped develop and promote the "Chain of Survival" concept to improve EMS response, early CPR intervention, defibrillation access, and coordinated emergency cardiac care. Eisenberg also promoted public AED access and contributed extensively to CPR and resuscitation research.

1987 The Citizens CPR Foundation was established as a U.S.-based nonprofit organization dedicated to increasing bystander CPR, public AED use, and survival rates from sudden cardiac arrest. Mary M. Newman, MS, of Pittsburgh, Pennsylvania, and Hans H. Dahll of Omaha, Nebraska, were among the key contributors involved in the foundation's development alongside EMS, resuscitation, and public health collaborators.

1988-1990 Mary M. Newman is credited with coining the term Chain of Survival in a *Journal of Emergency Medical Services* (JEMS) editorial. The concept was further developed and elaborated upon in *Currents in Emergency Cardiac Care* in 1990, emphasizing the importance of rapid recognition of cardiac arrest, early CPR, defibrillation, advanced care, and coordinated emergency response systems to improve survival outcomes.

1992 The "Chain of Survival" concept was adopted into American Heart Association (AHA) CPR and Emergency Cardiac Care (ECC) guidelines, helping establish it as a central framework in modern resuscitation education and emergency cardiac response.

1992 International Liaison Committee on Resuscitation (ILCOR) was founded to create international CPR consensus guidelines, to create a forum for collaboration among principal resuscitation councils worldwide. Basically, they help keep everyone on the same page globally, even though local science and regional practices might still have slightly tweaked differences. I didn't realize there were national and regional differences in CPR until researching this timeline.

1995 Widespread AED deployment in public spaces commenced.

1990s-2010s Emergency Cardiac Care Update/Emergency Cardiovascular Care Update (ECCU) was a biannual conference that was the rebranding of the Conference on Citizen CPR.

2000 Good Samaritan laws and AED legislation expanded throughout the United States, helping increase public access to AEDs and legal protections for bystanders attempting emergency lifesaving care.

2003 Dr. Gordon A. Ewy and colleagues at the University of Arizona helped advance and promote compression-only CPR, also known as hands-only CPR, for certain adult sudden cardiac arrest emergencies. Their research emphasized minimizing interruptions in chest compressions and demonstrated that immediate continuous compressions by bystanders were associated with improved survival outcomes in many witnessed cardiac arrest cases. approach focused on starting chest compressions immediately without stopping for mouth-to-mouth rescue breaths in certain situations. By simplifying CPR and placing greater focus on immediate chest compressions instead of worrying as much about rescue breaths, more everyday people were encouraged to jump in and do something when someone suddenly collapsed instead of standing by afraid of doing it wrong. The movement helped simplify public CPR instruction and encouraged more bystanders to intervene during emergencies. An American cardiologist and resuscitation researcher revolutionized bystander CPR with compression-only CPR.

2004 PRESTAN presents CPR training manikins designed to provide realistic, feedback-oriented CPR instruction for both healthcare professionals and community learners. Their manikins emphasized proper compression depth, rate, recoil, and user-friendly training features and affordability. This revolutionized CPR instruction for me personally. I love the click in the chest and the indicator lights of the classic PRESTAN manikins. PRESTAN introduced CPR training manikins designed to provide realistic, feedback-oriented CPR instruction for both healthcare professionals and community learners, contributing to the continued evolution of realistic and accessible CPR training experiences.

2005 Parent Heart Watch was established as a national nonprofit organization focused on preventing sudden cardiac arrest and sudden cardiac death in youth through education, advocacy, CPR training, cardiac screening awareness, and increased AED access in schools and communities. Formed by parents, survivors, and advocates impacted by sudden cardiac events in children and young adults, the organization helped expand national conversations surrounding emergency preparedness and cardiac safety for student athletes and youth populations.

2005 Mary M. Newman, back for the three-peat on the timeline, founded the Sudden Cardiac Arrest Foundation to help give survivors and their families a voice.

2008 Charlie and Karen Morrison formed MCR Medical Supply in Columbus, Ohio, helping support CPR, AED, and emergency medical training and equipment distribution.

2009 Cia McClinton birthed People's Choice CPR & Safety in Groveport, Ohio, with a mission centered around accessible lifesaving education, community outreach, and practical CPR and safety training, with a personal touch!

2010 Richard Price launched the PulsePoint mobile application to help connect nearby CPR-trained bystanders to suspected cardiac arrest emergencies occurring in public places. Utilizing smartphone technology and emergency dispatch integration, the app helped notify potential rescuers about nearby emergencies and AED locations, further expanding the role of community response and public participation in out-of-hospital cardiac arrest survival.

2012 Trio Safety, a company focused on CPR, AED, and emergency preparedness products and training solutions, was established in Birmingham, Alabama.

2018 GoRescue is born, from the union of Trio Safety and Stop Heart Attack.

2019 GoRescue hosts their first Lifesaving Summit.

2020 The first National CPR & AED Awareness Rally & March was held in Washington, D.C., where the event continues to be hosted annually. Organized by Ed Kosiec and Every Second Counts CPR, the rally and march brought together survivors, rescuers, advocates, healthcare professionals, and CPR organizations to promote public awareness surrounding sudden cardiac arrest, CPR education, AED access, and bystander intervention. The event emphasized the importance of strengthening community response systems and expanding lifesaving education nationwide.

2024 People's Choice CPR evolved into People's Choice CPR & Safety, reflecting an expanded focus on CPR education, first aid, emergency preparedness, safety training, and community wellness initiatives. The transition marked a broader approach to lifesaving education while continuing the organization's mission of accessible and practical community-based training.

2025 *The Wellness Pulse Podcast* was launched by Monica Stephens as a platform exploring CPR history, sudden cardiac arrest awareness, survivor stories, emergency preparedness, wellness, and lifesaving education. Through interviews, research discussions, and community conversations, the podcast helped bridge historical resuscitation science with modern public awareness and advocacy.

2026 *The Rhythm of Rescue* by Monica Stephens was published as a historical exploration of CPR, resuscitation science, emergency medical systems, survivor advocacy, and lifesaving education. Combining historical research, interviews, survivor perspectives, and modern CPR culture, the book was created to help preserve CPR history, reconnect people to the human side of lifesaving care, and promote greater awareness surrounding sudden cardiac arrest, emergency response, and community intervention.

Acknowledgments

First and foremost, I would like to thank God for His guidance, strength, and purpose and for the sacrifice of His only begotten Son.

I would be remiss if I did not thank my support system, made up of both blood and non-blood family, whose encouragement and support helped carry me through this journey. I would especially like to thank my mother, Cia McClinton; my church dad, Leonce Bowie; my best friends; my brother, Zachary, and his family; and my dearest Derrick McConnell for their unwavering support throughout this process.

I would also like to thank my church family and the many faith-based communities whose prayers, encouragement, wisdom, and support helped sustain and guide me throughout this journey.

I would also like to extend my sincere gratitude to the organizations, educators, advocates, conference communities, training centers, and industry professionals dedicated to improving CPR education, AED awareness, cardiac arrest survival, and emergency response worldwide. Special appreciation goes to the national organizations and advocacy communities whose continued work helps advance education, awareness, research, preparedness, and survival, including but not limited to the American Heart Association, the American Red Cross, Citizen CPR Foundation, Parent Heart Watch, the Cardiac Arrest Survivor Alliance, the European Resuscitation Council, the Heart and Stroke Foundation of Canada, the Australian and New Zealand Committee on Resuscitation, the Resuscitation Councils of Southern Africa, and the InterAmerican Heart Foundation. Additional thanks to the conferences, summits, and national events that continue to bring together rescuers, survivors, educators, advocates, and innovators, including the Cardiac Arrest Survival Summit (CASS), the Lifesaving Summit, the Heart to Heart Conference, and the National CPR & AED Awareness Rally and March. I would also like to recognize the advocacy foundations and awareness organizations working tirelessly to improve public education, access, prevention, and community response, including the Matthew Mangine Jr. One Shot Foundation, HeartCharged, Kyle J Taylor Foundation, In God's Hands Foundation, Huddle for Hearts, and Save A Heart. Special thanks as well to the CPR training centers, educators, and educational communities helping expand lifesaving knowledge and preparedness through hands-on instruction and outreach, including CPR Choice, Stress Free CPR / No Stress CPR Training, Health Force, and Sixth City CPR.

I would also like to acknowledge the companies, manufacturers, collaborators, podcast guests, and industry partners whose expertise, innovation, support, and dedication to emergency response education contributed to this work, including MCR Medical, PRESTAN, GoRescue, Laerdal Medical, ZOLL Medical, Avive Solutions, Defibtech, HSI, and Safe Life.

Finally, I would like to acknowledge the lasting impact and historical significance of Freedom House Ambulance Service and the many pioneers, educators, rescuers, healthcare professionals, advocates, and survivors whose work and stories continue to inspire future generations.

May this work continue to encourage education, awareness, advocacy, preparedness, and action in communities everywhere.

About the Author

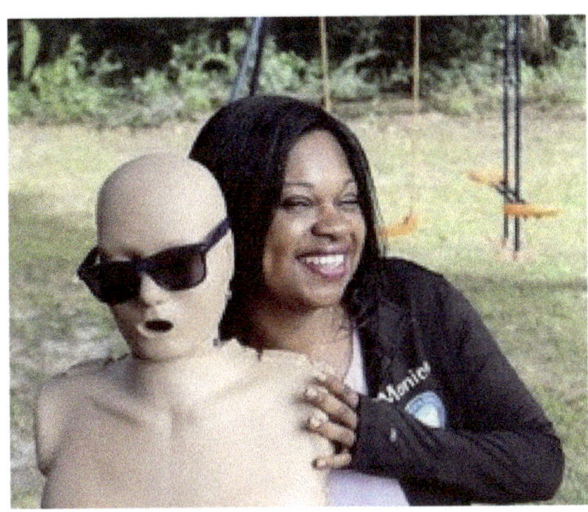

Monica Stephens, RN, is an educator, journalist, and entrepreneur based in Florida. She is CEO of People's Choice CPR & Safety, LLC, and host of the Wellness Pulse podcast, where she explores CPR history, sudden cardiac arrest awareness, survivor stories, emergency preparedness, and wellness education.

With Monica's background in journalism and public relations, she began teaching CPR and first aid in 2010. She blends healthcare education, historical research, storytelling, and advocacy to make lifesaving knowledge more accessible to the public.

Monica can be reached at monica@peopleschoicecprsafety.com.

www.ingramcontent.com/pod-product-compliance
Ingram Content Group UK Ltd.
Pitfield, Milton Keynes, MK11 3LW, UK
UKHW061955290726
14090UKWH00021B/1238

9 798894 201047